What others are saying about
Yoga in No Time at All

"After my heart transplant I tried the traditional methods of cardiovascular and weight training to regain my strength. No matter how hard I tried it wasn't helping. I then turned to yoga and almost immediately felt positive results. It seemed as if the yoga worked from within rather than merely on the surface. Matters of health are not something we should work on occasionally, but something that should become a lifestyle. The poses in *Yoga in No Time at All* are a clever yet elegant way to turn this practice into a lifestyle."

—*Kelly Perkins, Author of* The Climb of My Life:
Scaling Mountains with a Borrowed Heart

"As you flip through *Yoga in No Time at All* you may surmise that Joel is only offering us simple stretching exercises. In reality he is providing ways to bring the fullest depth of yoga, an integration of body, mind, breath, and a sense of something higher than ourselves into any given moment of our busy lives. His gentle and user-friendly approach will invite you to come back again and again. A delightful and practical book!"

—*Amanda McMaine, ERYT, MA Kinesiology,
Director of Yoga Teacher Training, Lexington Healing Arts Academy*

"*Yoga in No Time at All* provides creative ways to intersperse brief 'islands of yoga' into our daily lives. Whether you are just beginning or are an experienced practitioner, you will find something valuable in this book. Once you begin to experience these wonderful ways to take yoga 'off the mat' you will realize that the possibilities are endless! These 'islands of peace' allow us to become more in tune with the yearning in our mind and body to stretch and move on a regular basis."

—*Leslie Phillips, PhD, Yoga Instructor*

"*Yoga in No Time at All* educates us on small and easy ways to incorporate yoga into our daily life. There is a misconception that you must spend hours on your yoga mat to reap the benefits—and that simply isn't true. Joel has put a yogic twist on ordinary daily activities such as brushing your teeth and putting socks on. This is valuable information I can easily share with the students at my yoga studio. I am grateful for a book that is unlike any other yoga resource available!"

—*Sharon Tessandori, RYT, MS, Owner of Barefoot Works Yoga, Director of Teacher Training*

"I often hear my patients say they don't have time to exercise. Now there is no excuse! *Yoga in No Time at All* incorporates exercise into everyday life to improve health and mindfulness."

—*Margot van Eck, MS, PT, OCS, Bauman Physical Therapy*

Yoga in No Time at All

Joel DiGirolamo

YOGA
in no time at all

How to practice yoga in your **daily life** for
improved flexibility of mind and body

Joel DiGirolamo

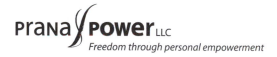

Prana POWER LLC
Freedom through personal empowerment

www.pranapower.com

Lexington, Kentucky USA

Published by PranaPower, LLC, 543 Laketower Dr., Suite 118, Lexington, KY 40502
Cover design and book layout by Noe Design, Lexington, KY USA
All asana photos are by Tim Collins and are reproduced with permission.

If you would like to purchase large quantities or a custom version of this book for your organization please contact the author directly.

Publisher's Cataloging-in-Publication
(Provided by Quality Books, Inc.)

DiGirolamo, Joel.
    Yoga in no time at all : how to practice yoga in your daily life for improved flexibility of your mind and body / Joel DiGirolamo.
      p. cm.
    Includes bibliographical references and index.
    LCCN 2009900682
    ISBN-13: 978-0-9770884-6-1
    ISBN-10: 0-9770884-6-4

    1. Hatha yoga.   I. Title.

RA781.7.D545 2009   613.7'046
                     QBI09-200021

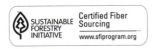

SUSTAINABLE FORESTRY INITIATIVE
Certified Fiber Sourcing
www.sfiprogram.org

Dedicated to Karen and all my fellow yogis.
I am grateful for your inspiration.

Our moments in this lifetime are numbered.

Meditate on each one of those moments.

Observe yourself in each moment.

Savor each moment.

Find love in each moment.

Feel peace in each moment.

Contents

List of Illustrations ix
Preface xi
Acknowledgments xiii

Introduction
    Intention 3
    Yoga 6
    Breath 8
    Computer Users 9
    Dividing Attention 9
    A Final Note 10

Asanas
    An Introduction to the Asanas 13

    Bathroom
    Shave Asana 17
    Brush Asana 21
    Brushing Forward Dog Asana 24
    Brushing Pigeon Asana 26
    Revolved Brush Asana 28
    Armpit Scrub Asana 32
    Towel Asana 34
    Prayer Asana 38
    The Rack Asana 40

    Bedroom
    Sock Asana 45
    Bed Asana I 47
    Bed Asana II 48
    Bed Asana III 50
    Sleep Asana I 52
    Sleep Asana II 53

    Kitchen
    Dishwashing Asana 57
    Dishwashing Tree Asana 59

Anywhere in the Home
Pet Asana I   63
Pet Asana II   65
Shoe Tie Asana   67
Phone Asana   69
Pick It Out Asana I   72
Pick It Out Asana II   75

At Work
Chair Asana I   80
Chair Asana II   82
Chair Asana III   84
Revolved Chair Asana III   86
Chair Asana IV   88
Chair Asana V   90
Chair Asana VI   92
Grounding Asana   94
Neck Tilt Asana I   97
Neck Tilt Asana II   99
Neck Tilt Asana III   99
Workstation Ergonomics   100
Break-Time Series   104

Driving
Drive Asana   113
Stoplight Asana   114
Filler-up Asana I   117
Filler-up Asana II   119

Shopping
Waiting Asana   123

Anywhere
Meditating on Each Moment   129

Contribute a Pose   131
Table of Difficulty Levels and Time
     Sorted by Time   133
     Sorted by Difficulty   134
Balancing Poses   134
References   135
Glossary of Anatomical Parts   137
Index   141

List of Illustrations

Bathroom

Shave Asana, right leg up 17
 left leg up 19
 right leg up, arm wrapped 20
Brushing without intention 21
Brush Asana, with intention 22
Brushing Forward
 Dog Asana 24
Brushing Pigeon Asana 26
Revolved Brush Asana,
 arm outstretched 28
Revolved Brush Asana,
 arm across the body 31
Armpit Scrub Asana 32
Towel Asana 34
 side view 36
 without the towel 37
Prayer Asana 38
The Rack Asana 40

Bedroom

Sock Asana 45
Bed Asana I 47
Bed Asana II 48
Bed Asana III 50
Sleep Asana I 52
Sleep Asana II 53

Kitchen

Washing dishes without
 intention 57
Dishwashing Asana 57
Dishwashing Tree Asana 59

Anywhere in the Home

Pet Asana I 63
Pet Asana II 65
Shoe Tie Asana 67
Phone Asana 69
Phone Asana with Neck Tilt 71
Picking out a book without
 intention 72
Pick It Out Asana I 73
Pick It Out Asana II 75

At Work

Chair Asana I 80
Chair Asana II 82
Chair Asana III 84
Revolved Chair Asana III 86
Chair Asana IV 88
Chair Asana V 90
Chair Asana VI 92
Grounding Asana 94
 with hands under heels 96
 with arms wrapped
 around legs 96
Neck Tilt Asana I 97

Workstation Ergonomics

Feet not grounded 100
Feet firmly grounded 100
Poor posture 101
Good posture 101
Break-Time Series:
 Prayer Asana 105
 The Rack Asana 106

Phone Asana with
Neck Tilt 107
Pet Asana 108
Grounding Asana 109

Driving
Driving without intention 113
Driving with intention 113

Stoplight Asana 114
Filler-up Asana I 117
Filler-up Asana II 119

Shopping
Waiting without intention 123
Waiting Asana with
intention 125

Preface

It seems as if our lives become more and more hectic as each year passes. We may cognitively know or feel in our bodies the need to exercise, but our list of excuses for not exercising seems endless.

And so I've written this book for you—you who know in your heart that you need and want to practice yoga, but never seem to be able to make time for it. I have created many postures that can be performed while you are doing other activities and many that can be done in a very short time without changing clothes. I also have included several postures created by others, which I have used with permission. If you have a posture that you would like to propose for a new edition of this book, see page 131 for more details.

During the development of this book several people commented to me that yoga done properly should be on a mat, with all of your attention in that direction. I wholeheartedly agree with this view. The difficulty is that there is a large segment of the world population who will not do that, at least not initially. This book is about meeting people where they are in their busy lives and bringing them a taste of yoga with the hope that it will improve their lives in some measure, and perhaps even get them onto a yoga mat.

Let me know what you think—good or bad. I am always interested in your feedback.

Namaste,
Joel DiGirolamo
(joel@jdigirolamo.com)

Acknowledgments

First, and most importantly, I wish to acknowledge the huge contribution which my wife Karen has made to this book. It would be quite anemic without her input, guidance, and nurturing. With Karen's "yoga voice," words flow out of her mouth like a fine wine, with depth, body, and that hint of raspberry and chocolate enveloping our souls as we practice yoga.

My personal yoga practice would not be what it is without the contributions of Karri Sandino. For many years, Karri and I practiced Astanga yoga together. As those of you who regularly practice with someone else know, these are mutually beneficial relationships. Karri has an innate ability to spur you on toward greater achievement in a gentle and caring way.

In one of those abundantly synchronous events, Karri agreed to edit this book. We are fortunate for this since she understands the essence of yoga as well as having the skill to hone a collection of words into an artful array of poetic prose.

Quantrell Cadillac and Good Foods were extremely gracious and helpful by allowing us to disturb their daily activities while we shot our photos. I'd like to give you folks a special thanks—and Billy, I hope I put the golf memorabilia back in place sufficiently.

I am grateful for the efforts of several people whose physical bodies are no longer on this planet. Through the cycle of death and birth, I began my practice of yoga at the age of 12 shortly after my grandfather died. As we were cleaning his house, I found the book *Yoga and Health* by Selvarajan Yesudian and Elisabeth Haich. With this book I began a clandestine yoga practice within the confines of my bedroom. The concepts taught by these masters precipitated both my spiritual as well as physical journey.

I have had many spiritual teachers in this lifetime, including Gautama Buddha, Paramahansa Yogananda, Jesus Christ, Lao Tzu, and Helen McMahan. Your contributions are woven into the fabric of my life, an integral part of each and every moment. I thank you.

INTRODUCTION

It seems effortless for us to slip into a mindless pattern of everyday ritual. The alarm shrieks in what seems to be the middle of the night. If we don't hit the snooze button, we unwillingly clamber out of bed, our body still full of sleep. We prepare our bodies for the day; we guzzle a cup of coffee (or two, or three) to slake our thirst for energy; maybe we eat some breakfast; we get the kids to school; and we haul our resistant bodies into our workplace.

All the while we are ignoring the voice of our bodies. It seems simple to close our ears to all of the ways that our bodies are speaking to us. Our knees may creak; we may not have the range of motion we once had. Our back may feel weak. We are winded climbing a few stairs.

Life doesn't have to be that way. It does not have to be reduced to simply moving through the mundane. We can change it. We can change our paradigm to create a whole new daily experience. Our motions do not have to be radically different, nor do we need an extensive amount of time. All it takes is a decision to change our intention.

Intention

By looking at your day as an opportunity to practice deliberate action, or a moving meditation, you can bring a new sense of awareness to your life. This sense of awareness can exist in *every* moment of your life—if you choose to practice it. The reward for this new awareness is an abundance of joy, a deeper, richer life, with a pure, pristine texture.

The concept is simple, but carrying it out requires persistence and concentration. Ask yourself: "What is my intention for the day?" Do

I want to "just exist" or to experience each moment as deeply as I can?

Think for a moment about your values and ideals. What are they? Do you value your health and your relationships?

Now ask yourself, do your ideals, values, thoughts, words, and actions all match? For most of us they often do not. We desire to be a certain way, to enter a certain state, but then do not follow through with the effort it takes to move in that direction. At our evolutionary best we are energy conserving creatures.

It is not difficult to change that, however. Spend just a bit of time thinking about what is important in *your* life. Write these things down on a small sheet of paper. Carry it with you throughout the day and add to it when you recall new things.

As you begin to settle in to the list, begin to observe yourself throughout the day. Are your actions consistent with your ideals and values? When are they and when are they not?

Are you ever triggered into reacting with anger or defensiveness? If so, what has triggered you and why? Is there some fear lingering in the background?

The concept of mindfulness, of watching ourselves each and every minute as well as setting our intention for each moment, is very powerful. It brings a whole new awareness to our lives, allowing us to see a new world in the same world. I am reminded of the famous quote of Marcel Proust, *"The only real voyage of discovery consists not in seeking new landscapes but in having new eyes."*

You can begin to observe your physical actions. Do you clench your teeth? They should touch only when chewing. Do you hold tension in your physical body somewhere? If so, bring awareness to it from time to time, take a moment to relax, and then continue on, setting an intention to prevent yourself from feeling tense.

Imagine yourself preparing dinner including local vegetables and other foods. You could set your intention on changing the environment around your dinner. If you have a TV or radio on, switch it off. Light a candle, prepare a cup of tea, pour a refreshing glass of water with lemon or cucumber, or a glass of wine. Look at the vegetables you're about to prepare. How were they grown? Where were they grown? Who grew them? Can you appreciate their color, shape, and nutrients? Can you appreciate the fact that you have them? Can you appreciate the people who grew and picked them? Can you appreciate the fact that you will soon have them in your body?

If you have a job involving frequent interaction with people you could strive to look each person in the eye; make direct eye contact, and feel a heart or energetic connection with them. It only takes an instant but can radically transform your outlook. For example, instead of pushing away someone with an acerbic personality or just labeling them as a jerk, ask yourself, "What is in the depth of his or her heart? What fears might he or she have? What trauma might he or she have endured?"

When an interaction begins to deteriorate, how can you respond mindfully instead of reacting abruptly or negatively? Think of situations that trigger you; then think through these steps:

> Take a deep breath
> Pause
> Observe
> Think of the best response for the moment:
>> Can I be helpful?
>> Can I be compassionate?
>> Can I be loving?

Often it's simply a matter of asking questions and exploring the other person's paradigm and history. Usually there is at least one fear involved!

As you begin to see each person and each moment in greater depth, your empathy, your compassion, your love, and your embrace of each and every single moment will swell and grow.

The words of Saint Paul come to mind: "Pray without ceasing." In other words, remain with intention, meditate on each moment, bring each moment back to God, Source, or whatever energetic force you feel connected to.

The concept of the Monkey Mind is often mentioned as an obstacle to living in the present moment. The Monkey Mind is an awareness that hops from topic to topic much like a monkey hops from branch to branch. When the Monkey Mind appears we are no longer conscious of the moment in which we are immersed. We have become detached from the deep still point within our souls. Keeping this concept in mind as we practice these asanas will allow us to enter them more deeply—both physically and spiritually.

Yoga

Some of you are probably wondering, "What in the world does all this 'intention' stuff have to do with yoga?" Well, yoga is not just moving through a bunch of physical exercises. While there is quite a bit of yoga knowledge in the West, we actually see only the tip of the iceberg.

Many yogic systems exist. The word "yoga" is Sanskrit for "union," which is related to the English word yoke. The idea behind yoga is to seek union of our physical and conscious self with the Divine, or God. This is called enlightenment, or *samadhi* in Sanskrit. Enlightenment may be experienced through several interrelated yogic systems including:

Bhakti Yoga – union through love and devotion

Hatha Yoga – union through mastery of the physical body, including the breath

Jnana Yoga – union through knowledge

Karma Yoga – union through selfless service and action

Kundalini Yoga – union by opening the seven major cakras (chakras) in our body to allow the kundalini energy to flow from our perineum out through the crown of our head

Mantra Yoga – union through sound, including our own voice

Raja Yoga – union through control of the consciousness, primarily through meditation

Tantra Yoga – union through a blend of physical and ritualistic practices, usually involving Shiva and Shakti

Yantra Yoga – union through vision and form, including art such as mandalas

Bringing us back to the purpose of this book, while many of us do not seek enlightenment, it sure doesn't hurt to get a bit of physical exercise! And—if we experience a moment with God, or the Divine, along the way, well, that's a pleasant bonus.

Within the Hatha Yoga system, several specific regimens or types of practice have been developed. Some of these are:

Anusara Yoga – a hatha yoga practice emphasizing alignment and an open heart with a spiritual and tantric focus created by John Friend in 1997

Astanga (Ashtanga) Yoga – a practice of 32 postures with a vinyasa, or flow, between many of them, popularized by Sri K. Pattabhi Jois

Bikram Yoga – a practice of 26 postures done in a hot environment developed by Bikram Choudhury

Gentle Yoga – a loose term indicating yoga focused on slow stretches, flexibility, and breath

Iyengar Yoga – a practice focusing on proper physical alignment of each posture developed by B. K. S. Iyengar

Jivamukti Yoga – a blend of vinyasa (flow), chanting, and spiritual teaching developed by David Life and Sharon Gannon

Kripalu Yoga – a meditation and asana practice developed by Amrit Desai and Swami Kripalu which emphasizes prana, self-acceptance, and taking what is learned in the practice into daily life

Power Yoga – a loose term indicating a vigorous, vinyasa-style yoga

Vinyasa (Flow) Yoga – generally a practice focusing on flowing from one posture to another, similar to Astanga, but usually not as vigorous

A practice of Hatha Yoga will bring many benefits including improved sleep, digestive regularity, mobility, and a healthier, more balanced appetite. As we age, we must consider three important elements for our physical health:

- Flexibility
- Strength
- Balance

Hatha Yoga is the only system that I have found which incorporates all of these elements in one practice. Hatha Yoga is considered to be a practice of both breath and postures, or *asanas*. In this book I will use the Sanskrit word "asana" and the English words "pose" and "posture" interchangeably. Related traditional asanas will be provided with each of the new asanas I describe. The asana names will be given in both English and Sanskrit. All Sanskrit words are written as provided by Nicolai Bachman in *The Language of Yoga* with occasional references to other common spellings.

What is fascinating is that as we awaken our physical body through the practice of yoga, other parts of us often awaken. In other words, this physical transformation can easily lead to some other type of reconstruction in our lives.

Breath

Although our lives seem to be filled with more and more tasks and activities, it is striking how infrequently our experiences connect us to our bodies, to the earth, or to the source of universal energy. Our breath connects us with this life force, and yet we can often observe ourselves holding our breath or not paying attention to it.

Yogis from India call the life force in our breath *prana* and exercises to promote breathing *pranayama*. As you practice the poses in this book observe your breath. Ask yourself, "Am I breathing deeply and fully, or am I holding my breath?" "Is my breath flowing freely?" "Am I connected with the source of life (*prana*) with each breath?"

As you practice each pose, notice your breath. Your intention is to feel connected to each breath, to allow air to flow freely in and out your lungs, and to sense that vital prana in each breath.

Our breath is a natural cycle that requires no conscious action whatsoever. At each exhalation you can become conscious of the toxins releasing from your body. Imagine your body discarding that last bit of stale air hanging out at the bottom of your lungs. If you can allow yourself to pause at the end of a full exhalation, you can relax and receive the gift of a natural inhalation, the gift of life and watching your body do exactly what it was made to do. That's a lot to think about in just one breath!

Beginning yoga students often marvel at the subtle intricacies involved in every single pose, including each breath. It may be difficult at first, but it can soon become natural and an act of honor and esteem to breathe in and accept the gift of this life force.

So as you practice a pose, connect with your breath, bring the energy into your body, and move a bit more deeply into it each time you exhale.

Computer Users

People who sit at a keyboard for many hours a day frequently suffer from a variety of maladies. I have found that many of the postures in this book can aid in relieving these afflictions. A dedicated section of short exercises for computer users is included here. If done every hour these exercises will greatly enhance your flexibility and minimize the harmful effects of this sedentary lifestyle or profession.

Dividing Attention

As you practice many of these postures you will also be performing other activities. This provides you with a marvelous opportunity to work at dividing your attention and not be focused solely, or attached, to an activity.

It may sound strange to talk about being attached to an activity but we do it all the time. We become so engrossed in what we're doing that we even forget to breathe!

Dividing our attention can best be described with an example. Suppose you are doing Brushing Forward Dog Asana as described on page 24. Here you are concentrating on brushing your teeth, as well as keeping your back straight, your heels down, relaxing your toes, raising the tops of your feet, and breathing. How in the world can you do all of that? The answer: with practice.

Here's a tip: first focus on your teeth for a moment, then your back, then your heels, and so on. The secret is to not get attached to any one spot.

This is where you can find the magic of your daily yoga practice. By quickly dividing your attention between many different views and elements, you will train your mind to more easily enter the state of the observer, or witness, as some people call it.

The witness state is one in which you can dispassionately observe unfolding events. Imagine that a heated argument is developing between you and a loved one. You become engulfed in the emotion and drama. If you are able to, take a mental step back and observe this altercation from a higher state. Said another way, by dividing your attention between yourself, the other party, and even your higher power, you can detach yourself a bit and handle the situation in a much more compassionate and loving manner.

This concept may initially be hard to understand, but as you practice it you can begin to improve your mental state as well as your physical being.

A Final Note

As you look through this series of postures, try to find the poses that fit you best and work on them first. For assistance, turn to the table in the back of the book; it lists each pose according to difficulty and time needed so you can scan the postures and make selections quickly.

Focus on the postures you can perform and find satisfaction and joy in whatever you can do. There is a saying in yoga that I enjoy very much: "The person who is doing the yoga that is most appropriate for them is doing the 'best' yoga."

I also believe in what I call the "Millimeter Theory." It goes something like this:

> Today, find joy in moving one millimeter deeper into one posture. If that is not happening, find joy in knowing that tomorrow you may move one millimeter deeper into one posture.

Remember, yoga is not about being able to practice every pose. Yoga is about making a connection with your body, mind, and soul. It is truly about the journey and not the destination.

ASANAS

An Introduction
to the Asanas

I have described each of the asanas in such a manner to help you understand how to get into them and how to get the most out of them—including the nuances that may not be so obvious. I have also listed the amount of time out of your day it may take you to perform the pose. Many of the postures take no time at all. They merely require a small effort on your part and an intention to maintain or improve your physical and mental health.

Each pose includes:

Time Required – Since it might be nice to begin with poses that require no additional time in your day, I have included a guide for the amount of time a pose may take.

Benefit – We often wish to target specific parts of our body to stretch or increase our range of motion. This element lists the general area of the body that will receive a benefit from the pose.

Difficulty – The difficulty of each pose is rated on a scale from one to five; a one-rated pose should be accessible to virtually anyone, and a five-rated pose may be accessible to only experienced yoga practitioners. I believe strongly that the more often you perform these poses the deeper you will be able to move into them and the more of them that you will be able to do. Be mindful not to push yourself too hard. An injury can set you back considerably, temporarily erasing any hard-won gains.

Muscles Awakened – Poses often stretch or strengthen several muscles. Knowing the muscles that each pose awakens can help you to focus your intention and maximize your benefit from it.

The index also lists the specific muscles awakened in each asana so you can easily find appropriate asanas if you wish to concentrate on a particular muscle or group of muscles. Some of these muscles as well as other anatomical descriptions may not be familiar to readers, and so I have provided a glossary of anatomical parts at the end of the book.

Description – A description is provided to prepare you for the pose, work yourself into the pose, and how to rest in the pose.

Traditional Asanas – Many times an asana demonstrated here may help with a traditional yoga asana. All traditional asanas referenced in this book are entered in the index. If you are looking for daily exercises that might help with Maricyasana (Marichyasana), look for Maricyasana in the index to find all of the asanas in this book that will aid in that traditional posture.

Variations – Some poses may be performed many ways, some easier, some more difficult, and some just for a nice variation.

Acknowledgment – For those cases where someone has contributed a pose I am including an acknowledgment.

To give you the best visualization of torso and limb positions, the models in the photos are wearing yoga-style, tight-fitting, stretch clothing. You, however, are not expected to wear yoga clothing during your daily activities. As long as you are wearing reasonably loose fitting clothing, you should be able to perform most of the poses.

Most of all—remember to have fun with these poses! Life is too short to pass up a moment of levity. See what you can do with a pose and don't forget the Millimeter Theory.

We all spend time in the bathroom each morning. There is no reason for us to spend this time without intention, without paying attention to our bodies. The following asanas illustrate how we can maintain awareness and intention — and move our bodies to enhance flexibility at the same time.

Bathroom

Shave Asana

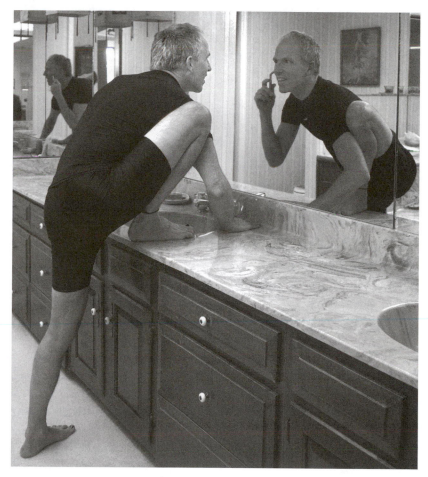

Shave Asana, right leg up

Time Required: 0 minutes

Benefit: improved range of motion for the hips

Difficulty: 5 (requires flexible hips)

Muscles Awakened: gluteus maximus, hamstrings

Description: Carefully lift your right foot onto the counter with the inside of your knee lightly pressing against your right shoulder.

Slowly lean forward, hinging at your hip without curving or arching your back. While practicing this asana, see if you can meet your gaze in the mirror and experience joy and gratitude for yourself and your life. Set your intention toward moving your collarbones toward the mirror in front of you, not downward. It is important to keep your shoulders level. Look at yourself in the mirror to check your posture. As you relax into this pose, feel your hamstrings and glutes soften and relax. Allow yourself to release more deeply into the pose as time passes. Of course you must keep your mind on shaving while performing this asana, which brings into play the element of dividing your attention. Switch legs halfway through your shaving process to give equal treatment to each hip.

Traditional Asanas: Arm Pressure Pose (Bhuja Pidasana), Big Toe Pose (Padangusthasana), Foot Hand Pose (Pada Hastasana), Sage Marici Pose (Maricyasana), Tortoise Pose (Kurmasana)

Variations: You can work yourself a bit deeper into this pose by using the hand that is not working (i.e., shaving) to wrap around the bent leg on that side. Place your hand at the edge of the counter to gently use it as a lever to work your torso forward if you wish.

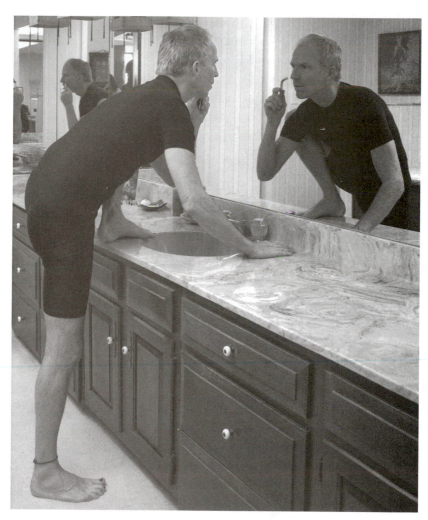

Shave Asana, left leg up

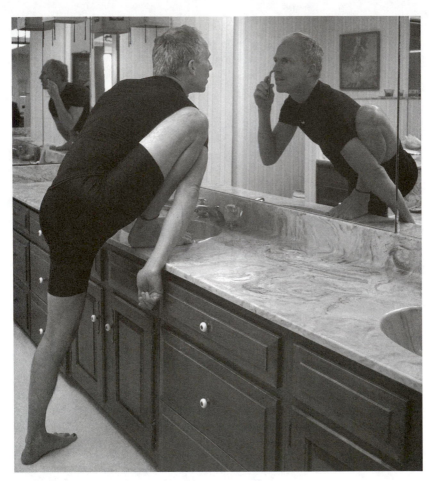

Shave Asana, right leg up, arm wrapped

Brush Asana

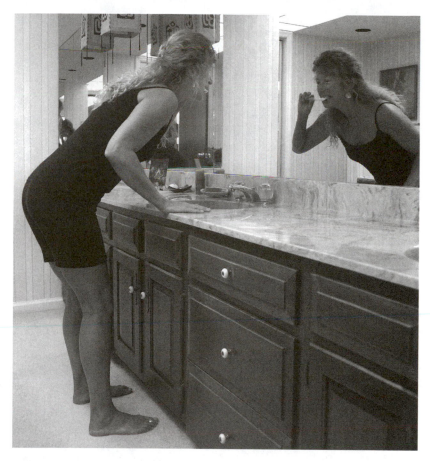

Brushing without intention

It is easy to allow our mind to wander while performing a mundane task such as brushing our teeth. As the model above shows, when not paying attention to the moment, to the activity at hand, our minds will wander and our bodies will lose their sense of purpose— that is remaining a physical, integral part of our beings. Here she is hunched over the sink with her back in a position that is likely to produce strain, and her feet splayed out a bit. Her intention is not set toward feeling her body and activating all muscles necessary to brush her teeth.

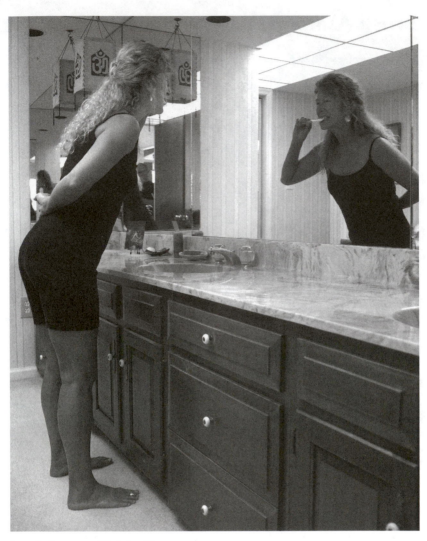

Brush Asana, with intention

Contrast the pose at left (Brush Asana) with the one preceding it.

Time Required: 0 minutes

Benefit: improved posture and presence

Difficulty: 1

Muscles Awakened: all muscles used to stand and perform the brushing action

Description: While this asana seems trivial, it is not. Begin by rooting firmly through the four corners of your feet (located in the inner and outer edges of the heels and the base of the big toe and little toe joints in the balls of your feet). Your legs should be erect but slightly bent, the abdominal muscles engaged and pressing toward your spine. Relax your buttocks, pubic bone tilted up toward your head, tailbone relaxing down toward your feet. This puts your pelvis into a posterior tilt, lengthening the lumbar spine. Reach upward through the crown of your head. Bring your shoulders back slightly to present your open chest in the mirror and engage your arm with the toothbrush. Don't let this arm droop. Enjoy brushing your teeth with intention! Allow your other arm to relax, letting it dangle toward the floor or resting gently above the back of your pelvis. Continue to breathe and divide your attention between brushing your teeth and keeping track of all elements of this posture. If you are doing this and not letting the Monkey Mind wander, you can get in a quick two minute meditation before beginning the day each morning!

Traditional Asanas: Equal Standing Pose or Mountain Pose (Samasthiti or Tadasana)

Brushing Forward Dog Asana

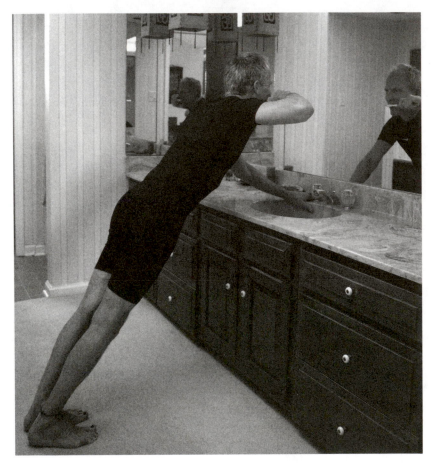

Brushing Forward Dog Asana

Time Required: 0 minutes

Benefit: lengthened calf muscles, aides in bending forward

Difficulty: 1

Muscles Awakened: gastrocnemius, soleus

Description: Place your feet back as far as you comfortably can, root down through the balls of your feet and lean forward, placing your hand against a faucet, sink or backsplash to support yourself. Gently lift the tops of your feet to deepen the stretch. As you breath, feel your calf muscles relax just a bit more on each exhalation. Bring attention to your toes. Relax your toes, ensuring that they are not digging into the floor. You will want to find a balance for how far back you place your feet. Locating them too far back will create too much tension in your calves and Achilles tendon. Placing them too far forward prevents you from gaining the optimal amount of stretch from this posture. If you are fortunate to have a patterned floor, once you have found a good location for your feet, you should have no problem quickly placing them in the optimal location each time.

Traditional Asanas: Downward Facing Dog Pose (Adho Mukha Svanasana)

Variations: Slightly bending each knee alternately will put a bit more pressure in the opposite leg, giving it an increased stretch.

Brushing Pigeon Asana

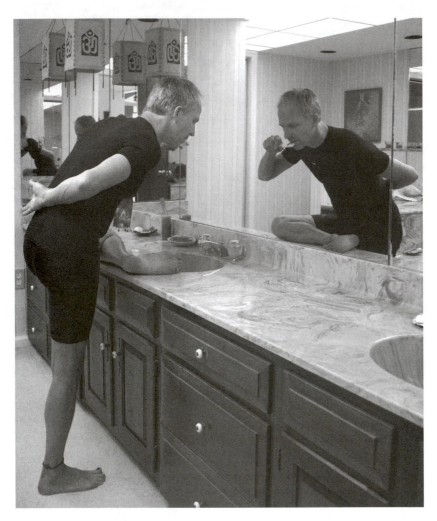

Brushing Pigeon Asana

Time Required: 0 minutes

Benefit: hip opening

Difficulty: 3

Muscles Awakened: pectineus, tensor fasciae latae (TFL)

Description: Stand in front of the sink and root down firmly through one of your feet. Raise the opposite foot and lift it onto the counter, placing the lower leg parallel with the front edge. Keep your abdomen back from your heel about a hand-width. Inhale, exhale, and slowly bend over the sink as much as you feel comfortable. Exchange feet about halfway through.

Traditional Asanas: Bound Angle Pose (Baddha Konasana), Half Bound Lotus Back Stretched Out Pose (Ardha Baddha Padma Pascimottanasana), Lotus Pose (Padmasana)

Acknowledgment: Barb Pfeifle, Lexington, KY USA

It is a paradox that by adding an activity during our teeth brushing ritual that we lose something—

our chattering mind.

Revolved Brush Asana

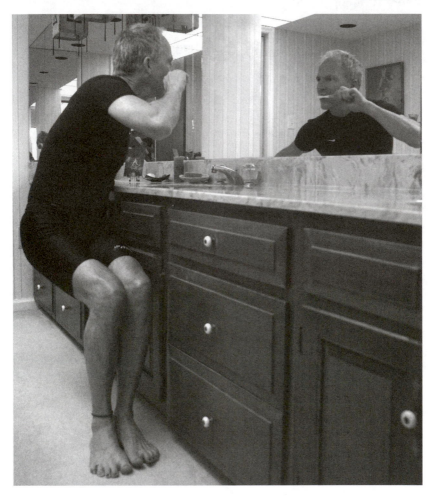

Revolved Brush Asana, arm outstretched

Time Required: 0 minutes

Benefit: improved back flexibility and increased back, quadricep, and gluteal strength

Difficulty: 4

Muscles Awakened: deltoids, gluteus maximus, internal obliques, latissimus dorsi, pectoralis, quadriceps, triceps

Description: For the description of this asana, I will assume that you are brushing your teeth with your right hand and will begin with your feet facing to the right. Left-handed folks will simply need to reverse right and left in all of the directions. Note that in the photo for the second part of this asana the model has moved the toothbrush to his left hand. This was done in order to clearly depict the asana in the photo.

Place your feet a short distance to the right of the sink, parallel to the counter. When you bend down, the center of your torso should be aligned with the center of the sink. Firmly plant the four corners of your feet (located in the inner and outer edges of the heels and base of the big toe and little toe joints in the balls of your feet). Stretch your left arm out and grasp the edge of the counter. Hinge at your hips and knees, bending down so that your thighs are parallel to the floor, lower legs and torso vertical. Your left arm should be extended outward, your hand grounded through the counter to support your torso. Ensure that your thighs are parallel to the counter, your pelvis level with the floor. As you twist, the side of your pelvis away from the counter will want to rise, moving into the twist. Concentrate on holding this side of your pelvis down, breathe deeply and with each exhalation, feel your body enter the twist a bit more. Extend through the crown, allow your tailbone to relax downward. Lengthen through your extended arm, feeling the connection with the counter. Continue breathing and relaxing until you are halfway through your teeth brushing. Now carefully rise and switch your feet so that they face to the left. Once again firmly plant the four corners of your feet on the floor, grounding into the floor, sides of the feet parallel to the counter, thighs parallel to the floor, lower legs and torso vertical. Again, the torso should be centered with the sink. Extend your left arm in front of you and across your chest, your fingers pointing to the right. Ground your hand into the counter or grasp the edge, relaxing into the twist. Inhale, lengthen through the crown of your head, exhale, relax into the twist. Remember to keep the outside of your pelvis down and continue to breathe. Due to the deep twist, you will find that your breathing is a bit constricted as you perform this pose. The deep twist is beneficial since it constricts blood flow, massages your internal organs and improves the flexibility of the back. As you exit the posture the inrush of blood can flush out affected areas.

Traditional Asanas: Extended Side Angle Pose (Utthita Parsva-konasana), Extended Triangle Pose (Utthita Trikonasana), Half Fish Lord Pose (Ardha Matsyendrasana), Revolved Side Angle Pose (Parivrtta Parsvakonasana), Revolved Triangle Pose (Parivrtta Trikonasana), Sage Marici Pose (Maricyasana)

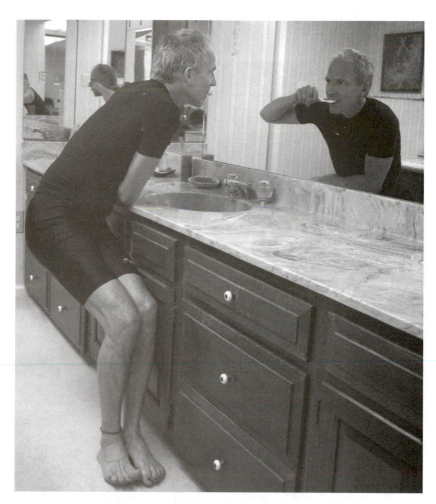

Revolved Brush Asana, arm across the body

Armpit Scrub Asana

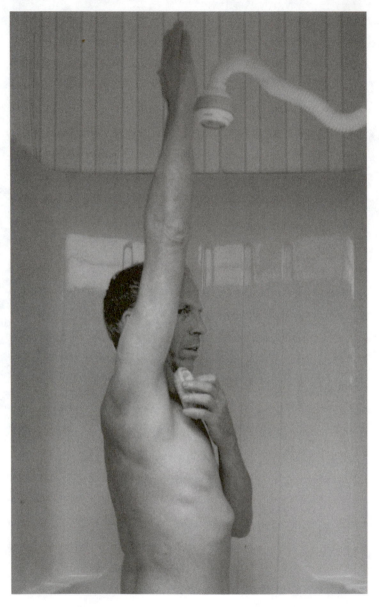

Armpit Scrub Asana

Time Required: 0 minutes

Benefit: improved arm mobility and range of motion

Difficulty: 1

Muscles Awakened: deltoids, erector spinae, latissimus dorsi, pectoralis, triceps

Description: Root down through the balls of your feet and extend your hand and the crown of your head to the ceiling. Breathe and allow your latissimus dorsi to lengthen while washing your armpit. Repeat with the other side.

Traditional Asanas: Chair Pose or Fierce Pose (Utkatasana), Sun Salutation (Surya Namaskara), Warrior Pose I & II (Virabhadrasana I & II)

It is symbolic that by outstretching
our arm toward the cosmos
we open a part of ourself that is
                typically closed to the world.

Towel Asana

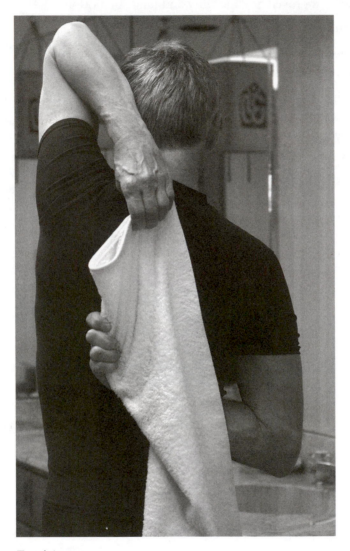

Towel Asana

Time Required: 1-2 minutes

Benefit: improved arm mobility and range of motion

Difficulty: 2

Muscles Awakened: biceps, infraspinatus, latissimus dorsi, pectoralis, subscapularis, trapezius, triceps

Description: Root firmly through the four corners of your feet (located in the inner and outer edges of the heels and the base of the big toe and little toe joints in the balls of your feet). Your legs should be erect but slightly bent, the abdominal muscles engaged and pressing toward your spine. Relax your buttocks, pubic bone tilting up toward your head, tailbone relaxing down toward your feet. This puts your pelvis into a posterior tilt, lengthening the lumbar spine. Reach upward through the crown of your head. Bring your shoulders back slightly. Grasp one end of a hand towel in your left hand with the excess flowing out between your thumb and index finger, draped downward toward the floor. Raise your left arm over your head, bending the elbow and allowing your hand and the towel to flow downward against your back, palm facing forward. Lower your right arm and then bend it behind your back to grasp the towel. Work your hands together as closely as feels comfortable. Breath deeply as you feel your triceps relax and chest open. You can use your head to gently nudge your upper arm back, intensifying the stretch a bit. Take several deep breaths and repeat on the other side.

Traditional Asanas: Cow Face Pose B (Go Mukhasana B)

Variations: This posture may also be done without a towel. In this case perform the asana as described above except clasp the fingers together behind your back, forming two "J" shapes to interlock.

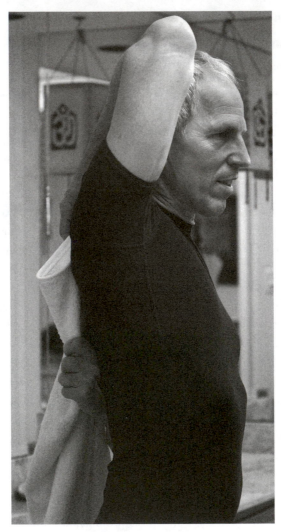

Towel Asana, side view

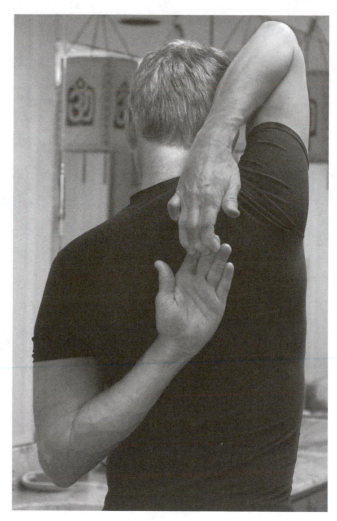

Towel Asana, without the towel

Prayer Asana

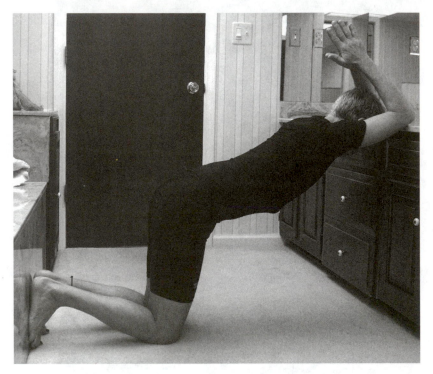

Prayer Asana

Time Required: 2 minutes

Benefit: improved arm mobility and range of motion

Difficulty: 1

Muscles Awakened: infraspinatus, latissimus dorsi, pectoralis, subscapularis, triceps

Description: Kneel at a counter such that three to four inches of your upper arms are on the counter when leaning forward as shown above. Root firmly down through the knees and elbows. Your feet may be flexed or pointed. Inhale and lengthen through your spine, maintaining a flat back. Place your palms together and allow your head to rest between your arms. Inhale deeply, exhale and feel your shoulders relax toward the floor. Inhale and lengthen from your elbows, through your shoulders, down your spine, and out through your ischial tuberosity (sitting bones). Continue this inhalation-relaxation, exhalation-lengthen cycle for five full breaths.

Traditional Asanas: Upward Bow Pose or Wheel Pose or Backbend (Urdhva Dhanurasana)

Acknowledgment: Leslie Phillips, PhD, Lexington, KY USA

A posture of humility that brings freedom to our body.

The Rack Asana

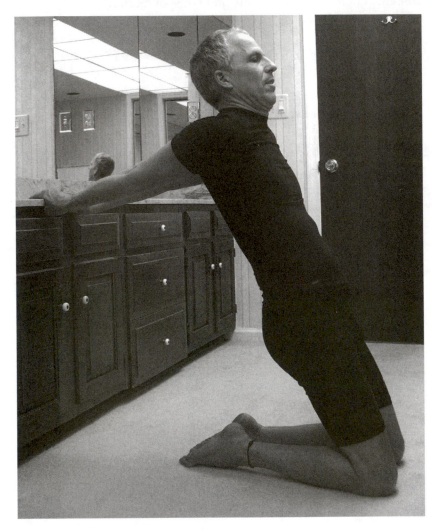

The Rack Asana

Time Required: 2-3 minutes

Benefit: improved arm mobility and range of motion

Difficulty: 3

Muscles Awakened: deltoids, pectoralis

Description: Kneel facing away from a counter with your heels approximately one lower leg length away from the edge of the counter. Place your hands on the counter behind you, thumbs wrapped under the counter, little fingers touching. Gently rock your body slightly from side to side in order to loosen the deltoid muscles. Inhale and lengthen your spine, reaching your head toward the ceiling and your pelvis farther in front of you. Since your hands are together behind you, this pulls your shoulder blades together, pushing your neck forward. Counteract this tendency by gently bringing your neck straight back, always lengthening your neck. Do not rotate your head. Continue to lengthen your cervical spine and imagine the top of your head lengthening up toward the ceiling. Continue to float your pelvis forward. Ideally your head, torso and upper legs should be in one straight line. Exhale and angle your pelvis out in front of you, continuing to roll your shoulders back to open your chest. Work your knees forward a few inches at a time if possible. Continue to inhale, exhale and move deeper into the pose as long as you are comfortable. When you exit this pose, do so carefully and slowly. Don't allow your arms to drop as they release from the counter. Allow them to return to normal at their own pace, slowly flexing and loosening as they return to their more natural state at your side.

Traditional Asanas: Spread Leg Stretched Out Pose C (Prasarita Padottanasana C)

Using free association, our bedroom conjures up a host of thoughts and memories, usually including relaxation, intimacy, and changing garments. While it may not be obvious, there are many moments when we can practice yoga in the bedroom, even while sleeping!

Bedroom

Sock Asana

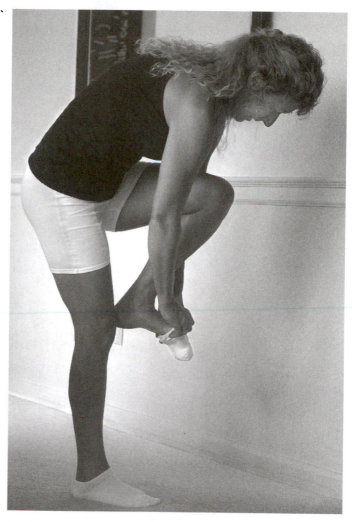

Sock Asana

Time Required: 0 minutes

Benefit: improved balance

Difficulty: 3

Muscles Awakened: gluteus maximus

Description: Grasp your sock, shift your weight to your left foot and root firmly through the four corners of that foot (located in the inner and outer edges of the heels and the base of the big toe and little toe joints in the balls of your feet). Hold this leg erect but slightly bent. Imagine the leg muscles hugging your bones. Engage your abdominal muscles and slowly raise your right foot, lean forward and pull your sock onto your foot. Slowly lower your right foot and repeat, raising your left foot.

Traditional Asanas: any standing pose, especially those in which you stand on one leg

Balance: a practice essential when
living in a universe of duality.

Bed Asana I

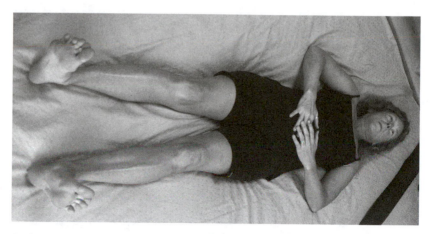

Bed Asana I

Time Required: 3-5 minutes

Benefit: increased body awareness

Difficulty: 1

Muscles Awakened: many muscles of the arms and legs

Description: This asana is almost as much about intention as it is about actual physical motion. When you awaken or when you are going to bed, as you lie there, feel your heels connecting with the bed, feel your calves, your buttocks, your back, shoulders, and head being supported on the bed. Become aware of your breathing. Alternately point and flex your feet (your toes pointed toward your head). Loosen and rotate your ankles. Bring tension in your quadriceps to slightly lift your legs. Breathe fully and deeply, feeling the prana enter your body, your ribs expanding and contracting on each inhalation and exhalation. If possible, raise your arms over your head and stretch. As you breathe fully and deeply, bring awareness to how your arms respond to each inhalation and exhalation. In the morning, sense your body opening to a new day. Think about what might be helpful for your body in this moment, in this day.

Bed Asana II

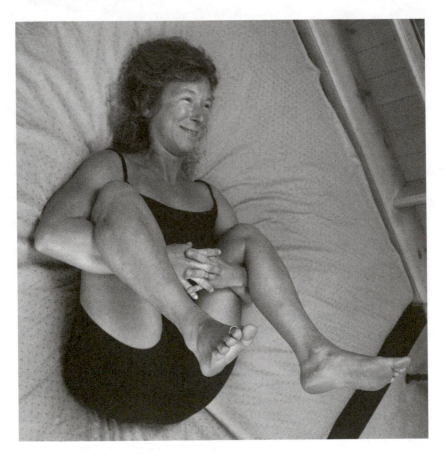

Bed Asana II

Time Required: 3-5 minutes

Benefit: decrease bodily stress, relaxation

Difficulty: 1

Muscles Awakened: erector spinae, gluteus maximus

Description: When first lying in bed, this is a good way to release stress from your day and to begin the relaxation of your body. Bring your knees in to your chest, wrap your arms around your lower legs just under your knees or behind your upper legs just above your knees and gently pull them toward you. Allow your gluteal and lower back muscles to relax. Become aware of your head and back being supported by the bed. Inhale fully, exhale and notice how your legs lower of their own accord. Allow this to enhance the stretch in your gluteal muscles and back. Relax while you breathe slowly and deeply in this position.

Traditional Asanas: any forward folding pose

Play brings joy —
   an essential element of a fulfilled life.

Bed Asana III

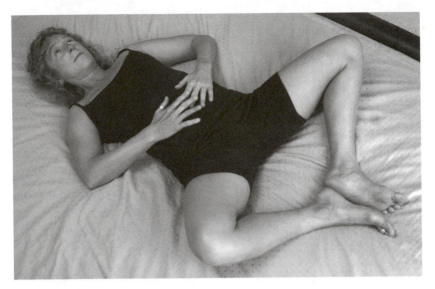

Bed Asana III

Opening ourselves physically
        —as well as emotionally—
    expands our being.

Time Required: 3-5 minutes

Benefit: improved leg mobility

Difficulty: 2

Muscles Awakened: adductors

Description: Lie on your back with your arms at your sides, palms up, or place them on your belly. Bend your knees and place the bottoms of your feet on the bed. Both knees and feet should be touching. Breathe gently, and on an exhale allow your knees to open to the side, the bottoms of your feet meeting, sole to sole. Bring your feet up toward your buttocks as close as is comfortable. Your knees do not need to be down against the bed although your intention should be for them to go in that direction. Take full, deep breaths and relax into the pose so that your inner thighs soften with each exhalation. Allow your back to relax and rest into the bed. Set your intention toward relaxing the adductor muscles on the insides of your thighs. You may want to occasionally place your hands on the insides of your upper legs to encourage them toward the bed.

Traditional Asanas: Bound Angle Pose (Baddha Konasana), Knee Head Pose (Janu Sirsasana)

Sleep Asana I

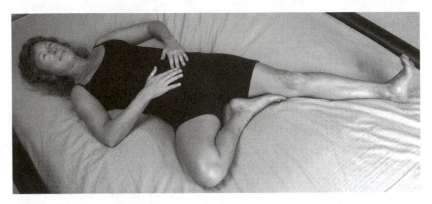

Sleep Asana I

Time Required: 0 minutes

Benefit: improved leg mobility

Difficulty: 2

Muscles Awakened: adductors

Description: Here is where you get to do yoga in your sleep! As you settle in to sleep, lie on your back with one knee out to the side. Gently place the sole of that foot against the inside of your other leg. Relax into the pose and allow your body to fall into a deep sleep, knowing that you will be doing yoga while you sleep. If you are sufficiently aware of your body as you awake during the night, switch sides and repeat.

Traditional Asanas: Bound Angle Pose (Baddha Konasana), Knee Head Pose (Janu Sirsasana)

Sleep Asana II

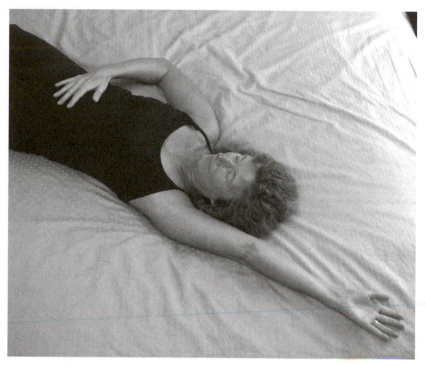

Sleep Asana II

Time Required: 0 minutes

Benefit: improved arm mobility and range of motion

Difficulty: 1

Muscles Awakened: deltoids, erector spinae, latissimus dorsi, pectoralis, triceps

Description: Lie on your back and gently bring your arm overhead to rest on the mattress above your head. If the headboard is close to your head simply bend your arm at the elbow so that your forearm is lightly touching your head. Allow your arm to relax into the bed. Consciously feel your entire arm relaxing and letting go. Imagine scanning your entire body with a wave of relaxation. Envision this wave entering your fingertips, flowing down through your hand, into your wrist, your forearm, elbow, rippling into your upper arm and your shoulder. Visualize the wave entering the fingers of your other hand and again down your hand, into your wrist, forearm, elbow, upper arm, and shoulder. Picture the wave of relaxation entering the crown of your head, through the inside of your skull, your eyes, eyelids, your facial muscles, jaw, and neck. Allow your head and neck to relax into the bed. Imagine the bed cradling and caressing your head and neck. Continue the wave of relaxation down into your shoulders, torso, and pelvis. Allow the bed to support your ribs, spine, and pelvis. Relax your abdominal muscles. Feel that wave of relaxation and unwinding in the top of your abdominal muscles, rippling down to your pubic bone. Allow this wave of relaxation to enter the tops of your legs and slowly ripple down to your toes. Become aware of the loosening in your upper legs, your lower legs, your ankles, feet, and toes. Once you have completed the first pass of this wave through your body, if you are still awake, begin again at your fingertips and allow the wave of relaxation to ripple through your entire body, relaxing every muscle along the way.

Traditional Asanas: Cow Face Pose B (Go Mukhasana B), Upward Bow Pose or Wheel Pose or Backbend (Urdhva Dhanurasana)

We sometimes spend hours in our kitchen preparing food or cleaning. The kitchen is a wonderful place for meditation. We can easily meditate while chopping vegetables or washing dishes. At each moment, with a singular focus, we can live it to the fullest, allowing ourselves to become immersed in the moment instead of letting our minds roam all over, or worse, letting them ruminate on trauma or difficulties in our lives or the lives of our loved ones.

Of course, while we meditate on each moment we can set our intention toward maintaining an awareness of how we are holding our body. Awareness is always the first step. We cannot work on that of which we are unaware. So use this time in the kitchen to become aware of your body and your intention toward how you would like to move it through your day or evening.

Kitchen

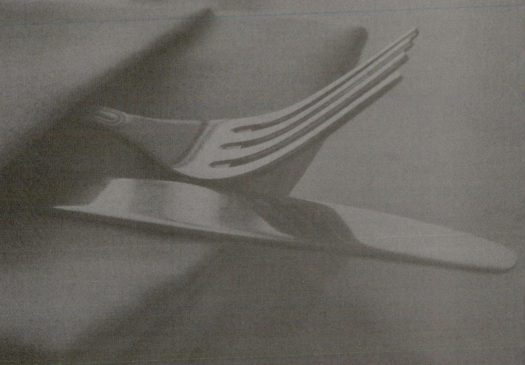

Dishwashing Asana

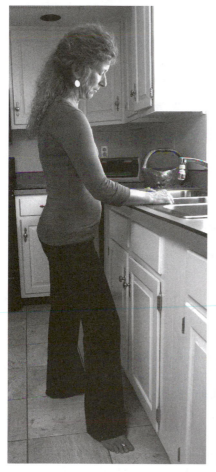 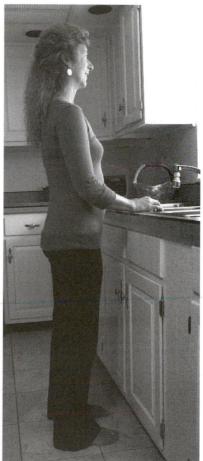

Washing dishes without intention   *Dishwashing Asana*

Washing dishes is usually a chore we do as quickly as possible so that we can get on with our day. With this attitude of being unaware of the moment or our current activity, we often allow our bodies to fall away from the activity as well. We can see by the photo on the left what happens to our body when our intention toward the activity is lost. Our bones move out of alignment, compounding our sense of not being present in the moment.

When we set our intention toward focusing on the moment, we can turn the act of cleaning dishes into a meditation. Gain intention in this activity by firmly planting your feet to the ground, aligning your ankles, legs, torso, arms, neck and head; you'll see it becomes easier to stay focused on each and every moment of the cleaning process, as well as to stay focused on the physical placement of your body. At the same time, your breathing will automatically become relaxed and free, allowing the prana life force to enter and depart from your body.

Through all of this, you gain greater awareness of what your physical body needs—and you honor it with the energetic sustenance of pranic breathing.

Time Required: 0 minutes

Benefit: improved posture and presence

Difficulty: 1

Muscles Awakened: all muscles used to stand

Description: As you wash dishes, set your intention toward caring for your body in that moment. Root your feet down firmly into the floor, wiggle your toes, and sway back and forth just a bit. Legs straight, but knees soft. Inhale and breathe into your hips and pelvis. Feel your lower abdomen expand and receive the gift of prana. Exhale and relax. Inhale and feel your chest expand. Exhale and relax. Inhale and feel your spine lengthen, your throat gently back and on top of your shoulders. Exhale and relax. Continue breathing and remain aware of the expansion of your entire body. Make this a meditation in dishwashing. Feel the fluidity of each breath as well as your sense of being alive and connected to the water, which is an element of the earth, and all that you see in front of you.

Traditional Asanas: Equal Standing Pose or Mountain Pose (Samasthiti or Tadasana)

Dishwashing Tree Asana

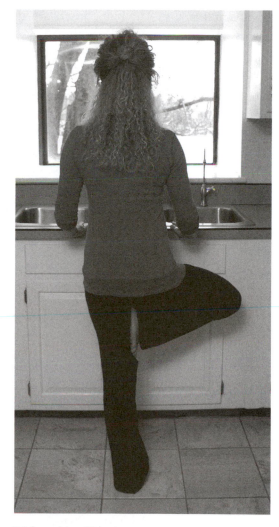

Dishwashing Tree Asana

Time Required: 0 minutes

Benefit: improved balance and range of motion

Difficulty: 2

Muscles Awakened: hamstrings, quadriceps

Description: Begin by rooting firmly through the four corners of the foot that you will stand on first. The four corners are at the inner and outer edges of the heels and the base of the big toe and little toe joints in the balls of your foot. Place your weight on this foot, inhale and lengthen from the bottom of your foot up through your leg, hips, torso, neck, and up to the crown of your head. Exhale and begin to inhale while slowly raising your other foot, allowing it to slide up along the inside edge of your standing leg. Bring it up as far as is comfortable, gently pulling it up a bit with the opposite hand if you like. Continue your dishwashing in this position, switching legs at some point in order to give the other leg equal treatment. As you remain in this position it should be easier for you to focus on the present moment, including the dishes and your pose.

Traditional Asanas: Tree Pose (Vrksasana) and any balancing poses

Acknowledgment: Barb Pfeifle, Lexington, KY USA

Surprisingly, there are many places and opportunities to do yoga — and bring intention, thought, flexibility, and focus to our lives — throughout our home. We are limited only by our imagination. When we think of ordinary, daily activities we frequently view them as mindless. Bringing yoga into these activities can transform them into something special and unique.

Anywhere in the Home

Pet Asana I

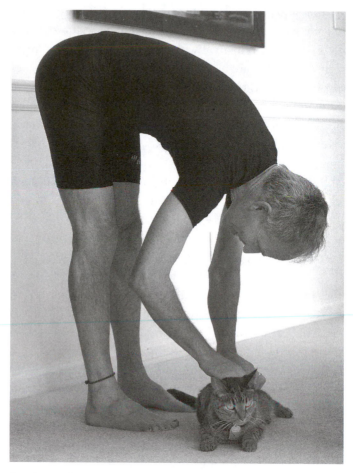

Pet Asana I

Time Required: 0 minutes

Benefit: improved range of motion for the hips, loosening the feet, and relaxation of the spine, shoulders, and arms

Difficulty: 1 (people with back injuries or osteoporosis should proceed into this pose with caution)

Muscles Awakened: erector spinae, gastrocnemius, hamstrings, piriformis, soleus

Description: Stand in front of your cat, dog, rabbit, or other animal and root firmly through the four corners of your feet (located in the inner and outer edges of the heels and the base of the big toe and little toe joints in the balls of your feet). Your feet should be parallel, hip-width apart. By placing the outside of your feet parallel to each other you are bringing your femur (upper leg bone) into a slight internal rotation. This internal rotation provides your hip with more freedom to move into the pose. Slowly and slightly rock forward and now backward. Notice how your toes become more active as you lean forward and how you can lift your heels slightly to loosen and massage your feet. As you rock backward, lift your toes to the sky and relieve the pressure on the balls of your feet. Rock back and forth several times to activate the muscles in your feet and to provide a gentle massage. Imagine that the outside edges of your feet are the bottom of a rocking chair, gently rising and falling. Now, standing straight and tall, allow your knees to soften slightly so that you are not locked into a hard and rigid stance. Imagine you are a culm of bamboo firmly rooted in the ground yet able to sway with the breeze. Inhale, engage your quadriceps and abdominal muscles, then exhale and slowly bend forward from your hip crease and allow your arms to flow to the floor. As you pet your animal divide your attention between the petting and your own body. As you inhale imagine your hip joints expanding, becoming more spacious and free flowing. Allow your complete spine to lengthen, from your tailbone through your lumbar and thoracic spine, up into your cervical spine. Let your head relax and drop toward the floor. Bring space and expansion into your shoulders and all of the joints in your arms and hands. Continue breathing, expanding, relaxing and petting your animal. With each exhalation you may be able to relax a bit more toward the floor.

Traditional Asanas: Back Stretched Out Pose (Paschimottanasana), Big Toe Pose (Padangusthasana), Foot Hand Pose (Pada Hastasana), Half Bound Lotus Back Stretched Out Pose (Ardha Baddha Padma Pascimottanasana), Half Bound Lotus Stretched Out Pose (Ardha Baddha Padmottanasana), Spread Leg Stretched Out Pose (Prasarita Padottanasana), Stretched Out Pose or Standing Forward Bend (Uttanasana)

Pet Asana II

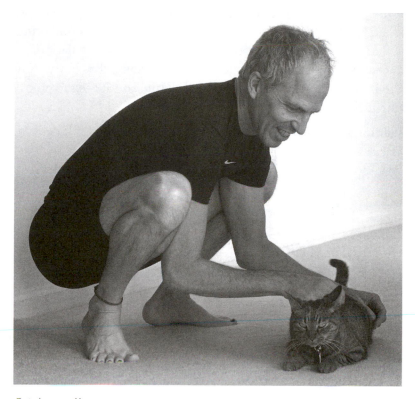

Pet Asana II

Time Required: 0 minutes

Benefit: improved range of motion for the hips, toe strength, improved balance

Difficulty: 4

Muscles Awakened: gastrocnemius, hamstrings, soleus

Description: Stand in front of your cat, dog, rabbit, or other animal with your feet open into a V, heels a few inches apart, spaced so that your hand with fingers outstretched may comfortably fit between them. Inhale, stand straight and tall, exhale and slowly squat down toward your pet. Your heels may want to rise as you squat, which is perfectly fine. Slide your arms along the inside edge of your knees, bringing your shoulders down as close to your knees as possible. Practice balancing on your toes if your heels are not on the floor. Continue to bring your shoulders toward the floor (or toward your pet) in front of you. Keep your back straight and bring your attention to hinging at the hip crease. On each inhalation, concentrate on lengthening your spine from your pelvis to the crown of your head. Breathe gently and deeply while continuing to enjoy bringing love to your pet.

Traditional Asanas: Noose Pose (Pasasana), Sage Marici Pose (Maricyasana)

Range: a span from lowest to highest. Practicing yoga will increase your range of motion, bringing freedom
to all parts of your life.

Shoe Tie Asana

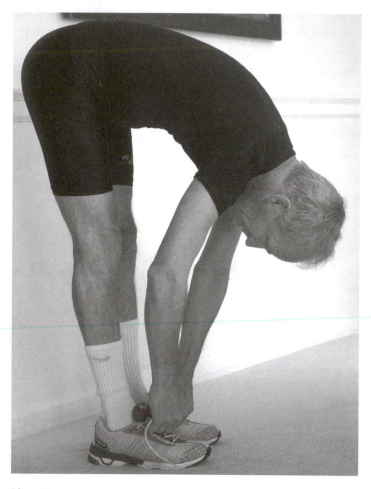

Shoe Tie Asana

Time Required: 0 minutes

Benefit: improved range of motion for the hips, improved balance

Difficulty: 2

Muscles Awakened: erector spinae, gastrocnemius, hamstrings, piriformis, soleus

Description: Place your shoes on your feet and root down through your feet. They should be parallel, hip-width apart. Inhale, engage your quadriceps and abdominal muscles, then exhale and slowly bend forward from your hip crease and allow your arms to flow to the floor. Tie your shoes while continuing to breath deeply and gently. As you inhale, feel your spine lengthen, your shoulders open and arms stretch out. As you exhale, feel your shoulders descend toward the floor just a bit more.

Traditional Asanas: Any balancing pose, any forward folding pose

Connecting with your body
while connecting with others...

Phone Asana

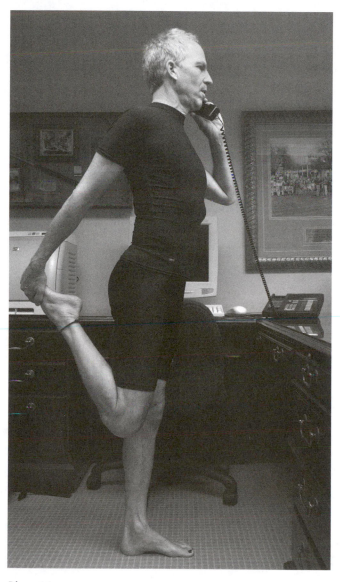

Phone Asana

Time Required: 0 minutes

Benefit: quadriceps stretch, opening for the shoulders and chest, balance

Difficulty: 4

Muscles Awakened: pectoralis, quadriceps, triceps

Description: This posture can easily be practiced while talking on the phone. I will describe this posture with the assumption that you are holding the phone in your right hand. If you are holding the phone in your left hand, simply switch the sides given in this description.

Root firmly through the four corners of your right foot. The four corners are at the inner and outer edges of the heels and the base of the big toe and little toe joints in the balls of your foot. Place your weight on this foot, inhale and ground firmly into the floor. Exhale, inhale, and lengthen your upper body toward the heavens. With each inhalation imagine bringing more space in between each vertebrae from your pelvis on up to the top of your spine. Exhale and begin to inhale while slowly raising your left foot, grasping the outside edge of the foot. Breathe deeply in this position for a few breaths. Notice how the toes and other muscles of your right foot wiggle to maintain balance. This foot remains active in this pose. Feel the stretch in your quadriceps of your left leg. When you are comfortable in this position begin to pull your left knee back toward the wall behind you. Keep your pelvis level with both hip points (ASIS, or Anterior Superior Iliac Spine) pointing straight ahead like the headlights on a car. In other words, do not allow the left side of your pelvis to rotate backward. Bringing awareness and attention to maintaining your left pelvis forward will also ensure you remain in the stretch. Continue to engage the glutes to pull your heel back. Relax your left arm and shoulder. Continue to breathe deeply in this pose until you are ready to come out of it. Repeat on the other side.

Traditional Asanas: Dancer Pose or Lord of the Dance Pose or Lord Shiva's Dance Pose (Natarajasana), all other balancing poses

Variations: You can increase the difficulty of this pose by adding a Neck Tilt at the same time. Of course this cannot be done while on the phone so it really becomes something other than "phone" asana, but we won't quibble about it. Grabbing your back foot with both hands will also increase the stretch that this posture provides.

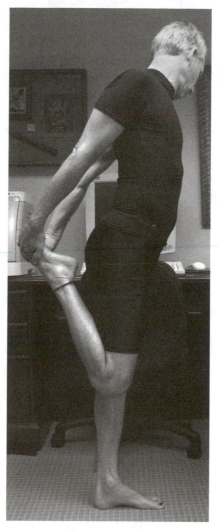

Phone Asana with Neck Tilt

Pick It Out Asana I

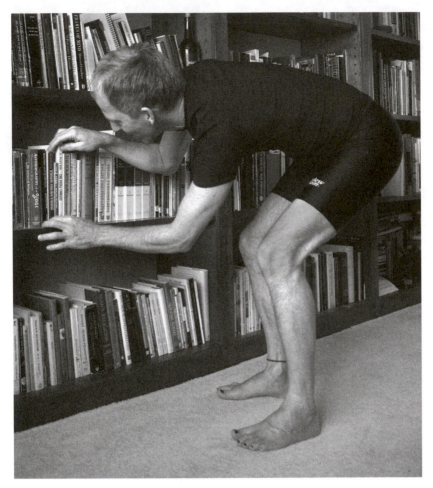

Picking out a book without intention

Looking for a book, CD, DVD, or similar object on a shelf can be a mindless task if we allow it. In the photo above, we see this person selecting a book without any intention or awareness of his body. At the worst, this can lead to soreness or injury due to poor body mechanics. Changing the paradigm, however, allows us to use this opportunity to do yoga. Let's see how this action can be used to stretch some muscles and improve flexibility.

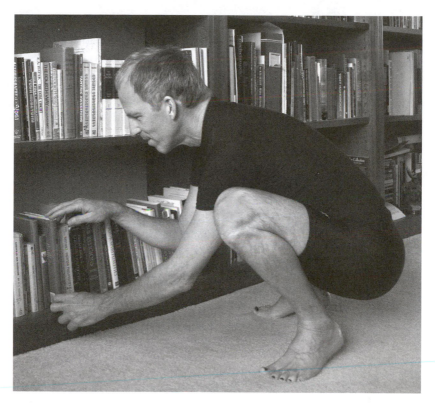

Pick It Out Asana I

Time Required: 0 minutes

Benefit: hip opening, balance

Difficulty: 3

Muscles Awakened: erector spinae, gastrocnemius, soleus

Description: This posture is mainly for selecting something that is low to the ground as illustrated above. Begin by standing with your feet shoulder width apart and in a slight V. Inhale, exhale and slowly bend down, allowing your arms to slide between your legs, elbows heading toward the floor. Look in front of you, not toward the floor. Bring your buttocks down toward the floor. Your heels may lift, and that is fine. As you are picking out your item, inhale and lengthen your spine. On your exhalation bring your intention toward lowering your sternum to the floor. Bring yourself into this only as deeply as you feel comfortable. When you are ready to rise inhale, engage your quadriceps, abdominal, gluteal, and back muscles, and slowly rise putting your intention in this moment to honor your body's ability to bring yourself to standing.

Traditional Asanas: Noose Pose (Pasasana), Sage Marici Pose (Maricyasana), balancing poses

Devotion: quite often it is not how much time we devote to an activity,
               but how we devote the time.

Pick It Out Asana II

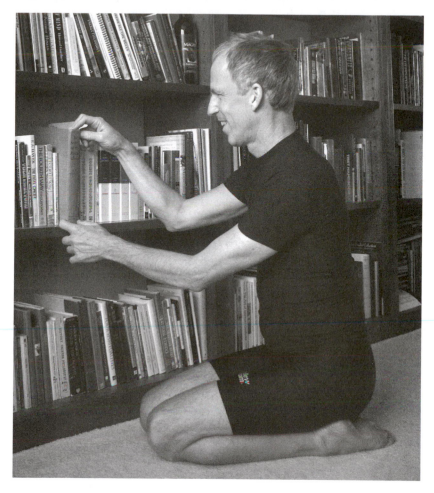

Pick It Out Asana II

Time Required: 0 minutes

Benefit: quadriceps stretch

Difficulty: 3 (this may initially be difficult for people with tight quadriceps muscles)

Muscles Awakened: quadriceps

Description: Begin by kneeling on the floor, your legs streaming downward out of your hip sockets, the tops of your feet as flat on the floor as possible. Slowly lower your buttocks onto your heels.

Traditional Asanas: Child Pose (Balasana), Hero Pose (Virasana), Oblique Face One Leg Back Stretched Out Pose or Three Limbs Face One Foot Western Intense Stretch Pose (Tiryan Mukhaikapada Paschimottanasana or Trianga Mukhaikapada Paschimottanasana)

Almost all jobs pull us away from our core, our center of peace and connection. If we are able and disciplined enough to take very short breaks we can feel a bit more expansive as opposed to compressed by the stress of a demanding job.

At Work

Most of us spend a significant amount of our time at our job. Unfortunately for our bodies, many of these jobs entail sitting for lengthy periods of time, often tirelessly pecking away at a keyboard.

In my experience I have seen that this frequently causes:

- Poor posture with a rounded back
- Slumped shoulders
- Forward head translation, which I call turtle neck
- Tightness in the shoulders
- Carpal tunnel syndrome (CTS)
- Tendonitis in the hands, lower arm, and shoulder tendons
- Pain in the muscles of the neck and scapula (shoulder blade) region of the back
- Repetitive strain injury (RSI)

The postures in this section provide relief for many of these conditions although it is vital that you pay attention to what your own body is telling you that it needs. For example, your neck and upper back may be sore or your shoulder tendons may be tight. While these postures will help many conditions, periodic massage and physical therapy may also bring significant relief.

Many of these postures can be done without taking up time during your day, however I am also providing a short "break time" series of poses that can be done in five to seven minutes.

Imagine the joy when work becomes play!

Chair Asana I

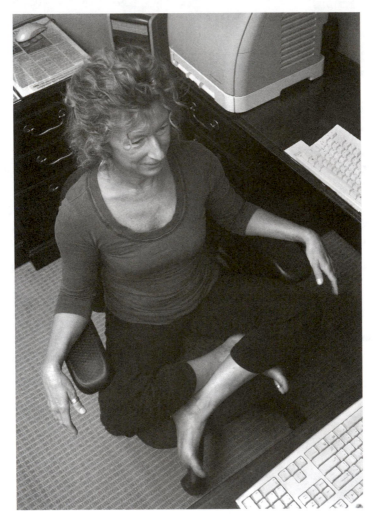

Chair Asana I

Time Required: 0 minutes

Benefit: hip opening

Difficulty: 2

Muscles Awakened: pectineus, tensor fasciae latae (TFL)

Description: Begin seated as you normally would and bring one foot up to rest gently beneath or against the opposite inner thigh. Bring the other foot up and tuck it under the opposite calf. Inhale and lengthen your spine, holding your back erect. Engage your abdominal muscles to bring stability to your core. Maintain this for as long as is comfortable.

Traditional Asanas: Bound Angle Pose (Baddha Konasana), Half Bound Lotus Back Stretched Out Pose (Ardha Baddha Padma Pascimottanasana), Half Bound Lotus Stretched Out Pose (Ardha Baddha Padmottanasana), Lotus Pose (Padmasana)

Variations: You can increase the hip opening by lengthening through the crown and rooting down through the sitting bones, lightly squeezing your scapulae together to open your chest, hinging forward at the waist and releasing your sternum forward.

Intention brings ease to effort.

Chair Asana II

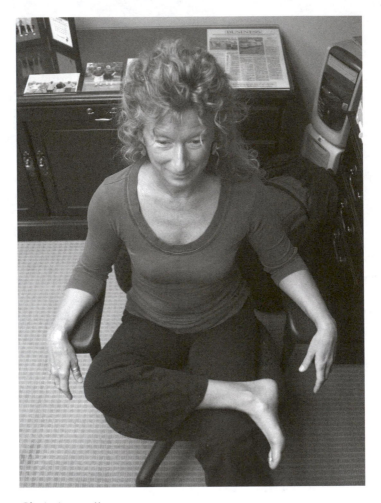

Chair Asana II

Time Required: 0 minutes

Benefit: hip opening

Difficulty: 2

Muscles Awakened: pectineus, tensor fasciae latae (TFL)

Description: Begin seated as you normally would and bring one foot up to rest on the opposite thigh. Inhale and lengthen your spine, holding your back erect. Engage your abdominal muscles to bring stability to your core and root firmly down into your sitting bones. Alternate legs so that each side is treated equally. This posture is easily done while in a meeting where a table hides your legs. Just think, no one will know that you are doing yoga while involved in a meeting!

Traditional Asanas: Bound Angle Pose (Baddha Konasana), Lotus pose (Padmasana)

Variations: You can expand this stretch by hinging at the hip crease and allowing your chest to fall forward. Raising the heel on the floor will also increase the stretch.

Chair Asana III

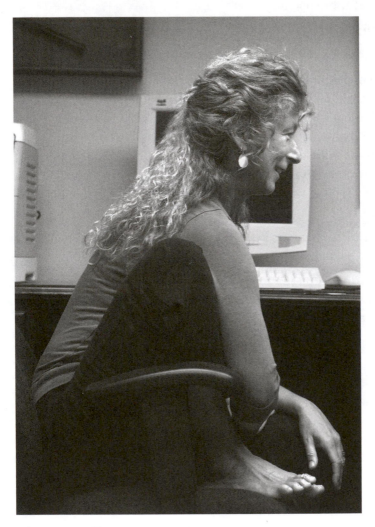

Chair Asana III

Time Required: 0 minutes

Benefit: hip opening

Difficulty: 3

Muscles Awakened: erector spinae, gluteus maximus

Description: Begin seated as you normally would and bring one foot up and root it on the seat of the chair. You can place your arm inside or outside the knee. Inhale and lengthen your spine, holding your back erect. Engage your abdominal muscles to bring stability to your core and root firmly down into your sitting bones. Alternate legs so that each side gets equal treatment.

Traditional Asanas: Sage Marici Pose (Maricyasana)

A paradox: bringing openness
by bringing together.

Revolved Chair Asana III

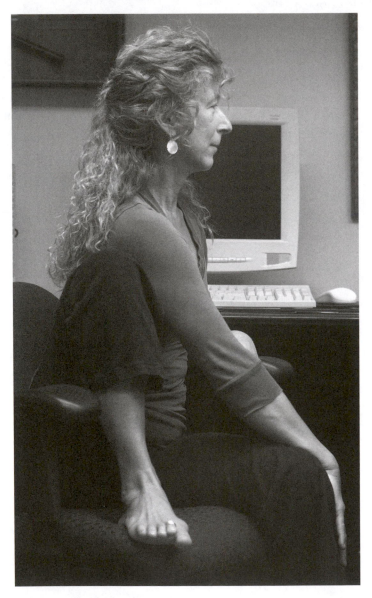

Revolved Chair Asana III

Time Required: 0 minutes

Benefit: hip opening

Difficulty: 3

Muscles Awakened: erector spinae, gluteus maximus, internal obliques

Description: If you are seated in a swivel chair, begin seated as you normally would and bring one foot up and root it on the seat of the chair. Rotate the chair so that the leg that is up rotates away from your desk. If you are seated in a stationary chair, bring one foot up and root it on the seat of the chair with your foot pointed out at approximately a 45° angle. Inhale and lengthen your spine, holding your back erect. Engage your abdominal muscles to bring stability to your core and root firmly down into your sitting bones. Remain in this posture as long as possible, maintaining awareness of the twist in your spine. Be careful not to overdo this posture. Alternate sides when you begin to feel your muscles speaking to you.

Traditional Asanas: Sage Marici Pose (Maricyasana)

Chair Asana IV

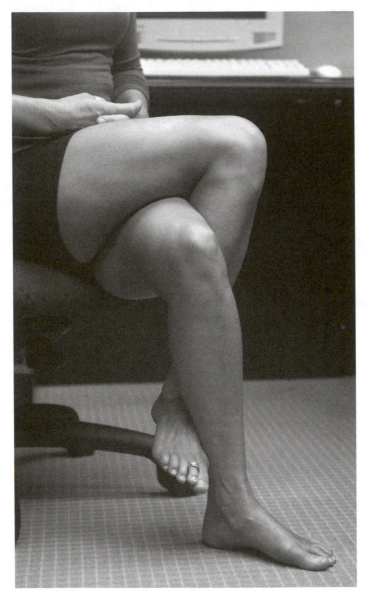

Chair Asana IV

Time Required: 0 minutes

Benefit: hip opening

Difficulty: 4

Muscles Awakened: gluteus medius, piriformis, quadriceps

Description: Here's another one you can do under the conference table. Root one foot firmly on the floor and bring the opposite thigh on top of the thigh with the foot on the floor. If possible, swing the foot of the crossed leg back, behind the calf of the other leg and wrap it with the inside of the foot against the calf. Remain here as long as is comfortable, then switch sides.

Traditional Asanas: Eagle Pose (Garudasana), Sage Marici Pose C & D (Maricyasana C & D)

Through stillness we create freedom.

Chair Asana V

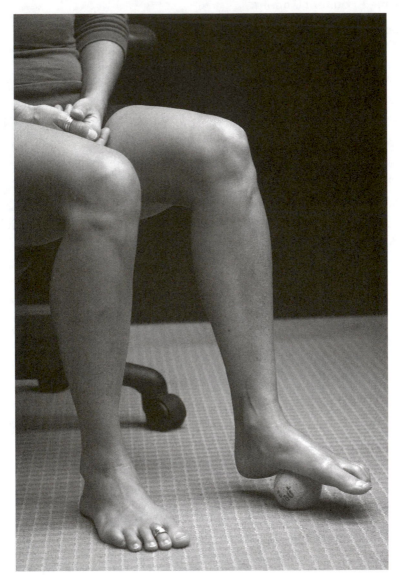

Chair Asana V

Time Required: 0 minutes

Benefit: relaxed feet

Difficulty: 1

Muscles Awakened: all the lower muscles of the foot

Description: This is really more a massage than a yoga posture, but I wanted to add it here since it is very beneficial and easy to do. Place a tennis ball on the floor and remove your shoes. Slide your foot left and right, forward and backward with the tennis ball under your foot. This will massage all of the muscles of the lower part of your foot. Ensure that you incorporate the full length of your foot, including your toes, ball, arch, and heel. Switch sides for equal treatment of the other foot.

Traditional Asanas: all standing postures

Variations: The ways to utilize a tennis ball for a foot massage seem almost endless. You can stand to provide more pressure as well as using a rocking motion rather than translating the foot backward and forward. When standing you can rock back and forth, alternately applying more weight on each foot, pressing the tennis ball down each time you place weight on the foot with the tennis ball.

Chair Asana VI

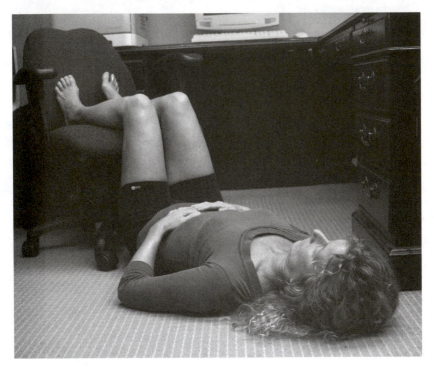

Chair Asana VI

Time Required: 2-3 minutes

Benefit: relaxes your entire back, shoulders, and neck

Difficulty: 1

Muscles Awakened: none, this is a relaxation pose

Description: Obviously, you will only want to do this where there is a clean floor. Lie on the floor with your buttocks near the front of a chair. Place both lower legs on the seat of the chair with your thighs vertical. Your legs should be as parallel as possible. Relax your low back into the floor, allowing the natural curve of your spine to loosen. Release your ribs and scapulae onto the floor. Relax your shoulders and neck. Allow your cervical spine to relax so that your neck can lengthen. Gently shake your head "no" to relax your neck. Inhale and feel your spine lengthen from the crown of your head down to your sacrum. You can stretch your spine just a bit further by planting the back of your head on the floor, lifting your shoulders slightly, tipping your chin upward, re-planting your shoulders and once again allowing your neck to soften and your chin to float down toward your chest. Ensure that your buttocks stay in the same location or you will find yourself inching away from the chair. Feel your thigh bones dangling from your knees as your hips relax down into the floor, creating space in your hip sockets. Remain here as long as you like, feeling your spine lengthen on each inhalation, relaxing on each exhalation. If you do this at your office, be careful that you do not fall asleep and get into trouble for sleeping on the job!

Traditional Asanas: virtually every one!

Grounding Asana

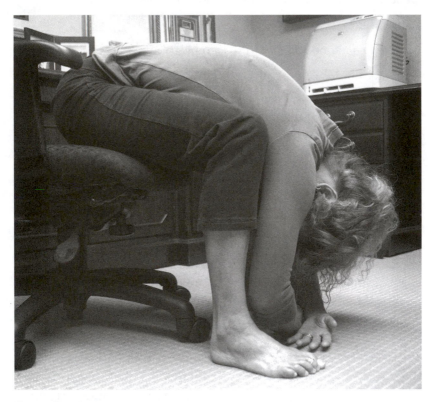

Grounding Asana

Time Required: 2 minutes

Benefit: improved range of motion for the hips

Difficulty: 1-4, depending on how deep you choose to go into the posture

Muscles Awakened: erector spinae, gluteus maximus, hamstrings

Description: Sit with your thigh bones in a slight V, lower legs vertical, feet in line with your thigh bones, firmly planted on the floor. Inhale, bringing space into your hip crease, lengthening your spine down through your sitting bones then up through the crown of your head. Exhale, engage your abdominal muscles and slowly bend forward at the hip crease. Bring your arms between your knees and open your palms to the floor if possible. If your palms do not reach the floor place books or some other object between them and the floor to give yourself a sense of grounding. Place your intention to bring your collarbones or sternum toward the floor. This posture is not about bringing your forehead to the floor. Bringing your forehead toward the floor will cause your back to round and reduce the hip opening we are looking for here. Try to keep your back straight, especially your upper back. If your palms are on the floor, plant them firmly, with your little fingers touching your big toes. Notice your breathing. If you are not fully into the posture, bend forward a bit more with each exhalation. When finished, engage your abdominal muscles and slowly rise up as you inhale. Resist the temptation to jerk upward and get on with the rest of your day. Stay present in the moment and honor your body.

Traditional Asanas: Downward Facing Dog Pose (Adho Mukha Svanasana), Sage Marici Pose (Maricyasana), Tortoise Pose (Kurmasana)

Variations: Placing your hands on the floor is not a requirement for this posture. You can use one or two books under your hands to bring the floor closer to you so that your hands can root down. No matter how little you bend, you will still receive a benefit. The second photo shows a variation where your hands are grasping the heels, pushing the legs upward for an added stretch. Here your hands are pressing up into your heels as you press down with your feet into your hands, maintaining the hinge at your hip crease. In another variation you can continue wrapping your arms around your lower legs and, using your upper arms, push your legs higher still.

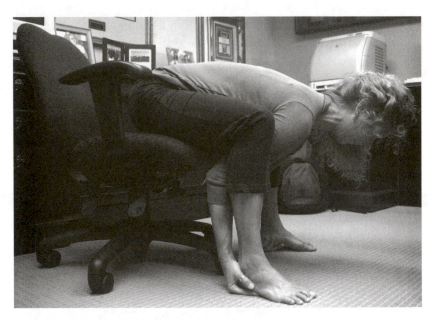

Grounding Asana with hands under heels

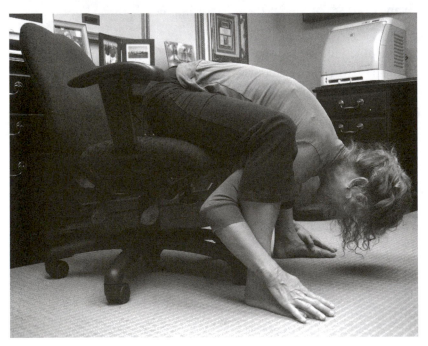

Grounding Asana with arms wrapped around legs

Neck Tilt Asana I

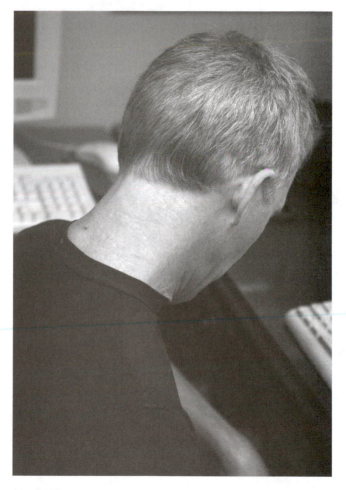

Neck Tilt Asana

Time Required: 2 minutes

Benefit: improved neck flexibility and increased range of motion

Difficulty: 1

Muscles Awakened: scalenes, sternocleidomastoid (SCM)

Description: Standing or sitting, inhale, lengthening your spine down through your sitting bones then up through the crown of your head. Exhale and translate the top of your throat back as if your head were on a shelf and sliding backward. Inhale and allow your chin to gently rise. Exhale and release your head forward, then slightly to the left. Now set your intention toward reaching the crown of your head away from the back side of your right shoulder. Inhale, exhale and allow your head to drop, relax your shoulders and allow them to float downward toward the floor. With each inhalation and exhalation allow your head to droop slightly lower, feeling the muscles in the back right quarter of your neck and the back of your shoulder relax. Feel your entire right shoulder flowing away from your head, opening your chest as well as your neck. Imagine your breath on each inhalation opening your right shoulder a bit more. When you feel that your right shoulder has stretched sufficiently inhale your head upright, exhale, inhale, lengthen, translate the top of your throat back once again, exhale, and allow your head to drop forward and slightly to the right. Repeat all elements of the asana on the right side.

Traditional Asanas: all twisting postures

Neck Tilt Asana II

Time Required: 2 minutes

Benefit: improved neck flexibility and increased range of motion

Difficulty: 1

Muscles Awakened: scalenes, sternocleidomastoid (SCM)

Description: Standing or sitting, inhale and lengthen your spine down through your sitting bones then up through the crown of your head. Exhale and release your head to the left, bringing your ear down toward your shoulder. Keep your shoulders level, allowing them to hang heavy from your spine. Release your right hand toward the floor, your fingertips lengthening downward. On each inhalation feel your crown reaching upward. On each exhalation feel your right side lengthening a bit more. To enhance the stretch, further extend your left arm outward, fingers reaching toward the wall on your left. Continue breathing and feeling the stretch in your neck. Repeat on the opposite side.

Neck Tilt Asana III

Time Required: 2 minutes

Benefit: improved neck flexibility and increased range of motion

Difficulty: 1

Muscles Awakened: trapezius

Description: Standing or sitting, inhale and lengthen your spine down through your sitting bones then up through the crown of your head. Exhale and slowly lift the base of your skull, tuck your chin and reach upward through your crown. Continue breathing, lengthening on your inhalation and lifting the base of your skull on your exhalation. Keep your chest open, your shoulders wide, and shoulder blades gliding down your back. On an inhalation slowly rotate your head toward the right. Exhale and lift the base of your skull. Inhale, lengthen, and rotate just a bit more. Exhale and lift the base of your skull. Inhale your head back to straight ahead. Repeat toward the left side and inhale your head back to center. Exhale, then inhale your head up to bring your eyes level with the horizon.

Workstation Ergonomics

It is important that our workstations have proper ergonomics for our individual bodies. Each one of us is built differently. Some of us have longer torsos, longer legs, etc.

The following elements are critical for a healthy body:
- Chair height in relation to the floor
- Chair height in relation to your keyboard or writing surface
- Display and keyboard or laptop computer directly in front of you
- Display height in relation to your eye height
- Type of glasses worn and their relation in height to the display
- Type of navigational device, such as mouse, trackball, or tablet

Begin by adjusting your **chair** height so that your feet are flat, rooting down into the floor. When your feet are not flat, you become ungrounded and your knee joints will tire and become stressed. If your chair will not adjust properly you can add a cushion to your seat or obtain a footrest.

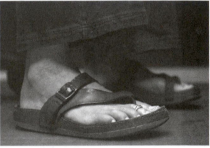

Feet firmly grounded

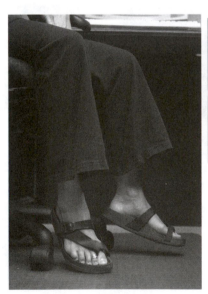

Feet not grounded

Once your feet are well grounded look at the relationship of your hands to your keyboard. Our hands are not naturally inclined to lie flat on a keyboard. Place your hands flat on a desk in front of you with your thumbs touching. Keeping your hands flat, rotate them so that your thumbs rise and your little fingers stay on the desk. Raise them to about a 45° angle. This is a natural position for your hands.

Keyboards may be purchased that allow your hands to stay in this position, thus minimizing stress on your hands, wrists, elbows, and all of the muscles in your upper arms. If you do find your fingers, wrists, arms, neck, or shoulders are tight or sore, massage and physical therapy can provide significant relief.

Your keyboard height should be adjusted so that your wrists are not bent up or down and that your upper arms hang comfortably at the sides of your body. If your keyboard is too high in relation to your shoulders, you will find that your neck and shoulders become sore and cramped from continually lifting your shoulders. If your keyboard is too low your wrists will become strained from bending

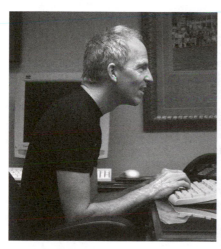

Poor posture

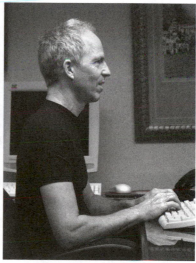

Good posture

backward. In general, if your forearms are parallel to the floor your keyboard will be at a good height for you.

If your keyboard height is not adjustable consider getting an adjustable keyboard tray or extender that allows considerable height and angle adjustment. Ideally you want your hands to stream straight out level with your forearms and wrists.

It is vital for you to place yourself directly in front of your keyboard and **monitor**. Placing your monitor to one side can cause substantial neck strain. If your keyboard is off to one side your torso must twist to place your hands on the keyboard. This puts considerable strain on many of the back, neck, and shoulder muscles.

The height of your monitor should be such that you can easily lengthen your spine and maintain a posture with your head over your shoulders. Your eyes should be looking slightly downward. If you are having to look up, you will strain your neck. Continually looking down will cause you to translate your head forward and down, causing turtle neck, as shown on the previous page.

By translating your throat back toward the wall behind you, your posture will improve. Imagine taking the portion of your neck just below your chin straight back, maintaining length in your neck.

The type of **glasses** that you use can also cause problems. If you spend a considerable amount of time in front of your computer wearing bifocal glasses, you may discover they cause neck strain because of repeatedly having to lift your head to look out of the bottom part of the bifocal. A good solution is to measure the distance from your monitor to your eyes and have your eye doctor prescribe full-view glasses that provide optimum focus for this distance.

Several types of navigation devices are currently on the market, with the mouse being the overwhelming favorite. Since these devices are used for many hours each day, they may tend to cause repetitive stress conditions such as carpal tunnel difficulties, tendonitis, and tightness or tension in the upper arms, shoulders, and neck.

Using a **mouse** can cause tendonitis in the fingers from frequent button clicking and tendonitis in the upper arms. If you become sore from extended use of your mouse, consider switching hands. It will take time to gain proficiency but you may be surprised how short the learning curve is. Once you have mastered using both hands you can easily switch from side to side, providing a bit of relief. A trackball is another alternative, although I and many others have found that trackballs have a tendency to cause tendonitis in the upper arm.

An excellent alternative is a tablet with a stylus. These seem to cause fewer repetitive injuries and are reasonably priced.

As you are working, notice from time to time how you hold your **shoulders**. Are they taut and reaching for your ears? If so, relax them, bring them forward and backward and up and down. Try to maintain this fluidity and relaxed state as you work throughout the day.

Break-Time Series

For those of you sitting at a desk all day, your body will get stiff and sore since your joints and muscles are not as active as they are intended to be. I highly recommend stopping once an hour or at least every two hours and practicing the following five poses. You can easily set a timer on your computer for this. These five poses should take only four to five minutes to complete. Hold each pose until you feel your muscles stretched to their greatest extent, generally five or six breaths. These short exercises will give you a physical, as well as mental benefit.

1. Prayer Asana (page 38)
2. The Rack Asana (page 40)
3. Phone Asana with Neck Tilt (page 71)
4. Pet Asana I or II (pages 63 and 65)
5. Grounding Asana (page 94)

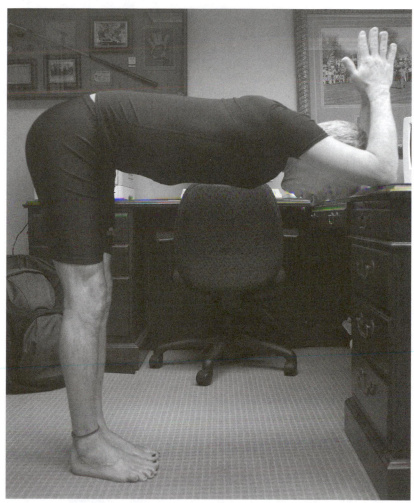

1. Prayer Asana in the office

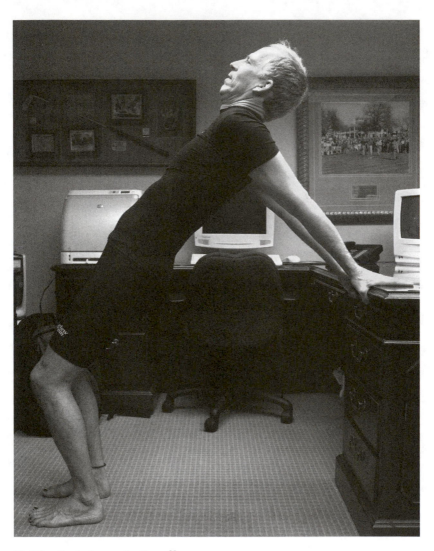

2. The Rack Asana in the office

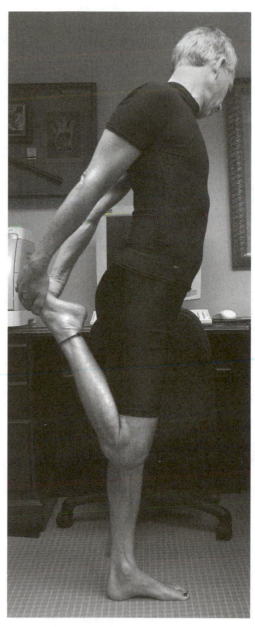

3. Phone Asana with Neck Tilt in the office

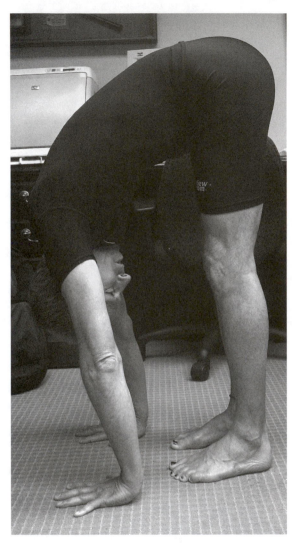

4. Pet Asana in the office

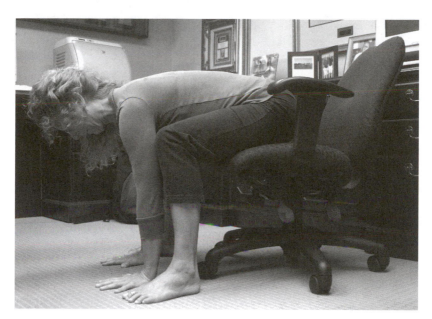

5. Grounding Asana in the office

Driving can be a mindless activity where we lose our self into random thoughts or it can sometimes be an intense activity when we are hurrying to work or an appointment. This will often cause us to lose our body awareness.

Driving

Drive Asana

As the photo below illustrates, we can often end up slumped down in our seats, and causing numerous physical strains on our bodies. Driving with intention means that we are aware of our body position and the strain we are placing on our muscles. By remaining aware of your breath and how your torso is positioned, you can easily maintain good posture so that your arms, neck, and shoulders relax during your entire trip.

Think of practicing yoga during your drive. Stay conscious of your breath and lengthen through your torso, shoulders, and neck. Relax your arms on the steering wheel and breathe.

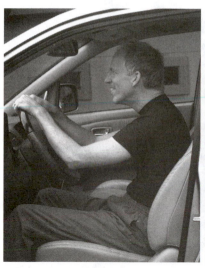 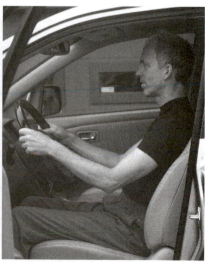

Driving without intention   *Driving with intention*

Stoplight Asana

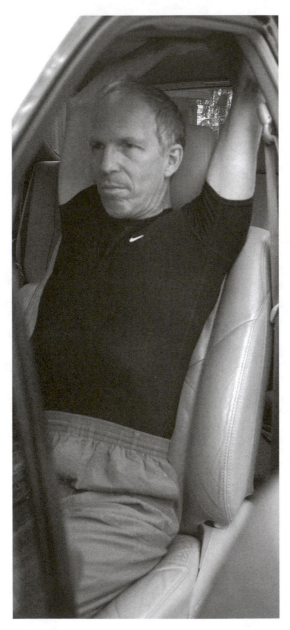

Stoplight Asana

Time Required: 0 minutes

Benefit: improved range of motion for the arms

Difficulty: 1

Muscles Awakened: deltoids, latissimus dorsi, pectoralis

Description: When you are stopped at a traffic light or in traffic, raise your arms overhead and behind you as much as possible. Place your hands firmly against the roof of your vehicle. Inhale, root down into the seat, lengthen up through your spine and all the way out into your fingertips. Exhale and allow your hands, neck, and shoulders to relax backward. Inhale and lift your sternum to the windshield. Feel your breath filling the back plane of your body, your entire torso expanding and lengthening. Exhale your hands, neck, and shoulders back. Repeat this pattern for as long as desired.

Traditional Asanas: Downward Facing Dog Pose (Adho Mukha Svanasana), Upward Bow Pose or Wheel Pose or Backbend (Urdhva Dhanurasana)

Gas Station

Filling our vehicles with gasoline can easily be considered another of those mindless activities. As you fill up your vehicle look around for props to use for stretching, especially if you've been driving for hours on the interstate or autobahn. Your vehicle, light or roof poles, and trash containers provide convenient props to brace yourself and stretch with these asanas. This will allow you to move from the view that filling your tank is a waste of time to the view that it is an opportunity to do yoga!

Filler-up Asana I

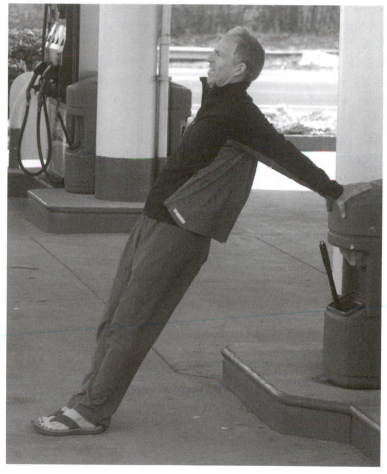

Filler-up Asana I

Time Required: 0 minutes

Benefit: improved arm mobility and range of motion

Difficulty: 3

Muscles Awakened: deltoids, pectoralis

Description: This pose is very similar to The Rack and can be done while your tank is filling. Stand with your hands behind you, little fingers touching each other. Place them on the trunk of your car or another sturdy object at the gas station. Slowly walk away while your hands remain stationary and your body remains straight from the knees up. Stop when your lower legs are vertical and when you feel that your shoulders are stretched to their limit. Inhale and feel your chest expand. Relax and allow your spine to lengthen. Exhale and relax your shoulders. Take a small step forward if possible, and bring your body straight from the knees up. Ensure that your neck, throat, and head are translated back and your spine is lengthened. Inhale and feel your chest expand and spine lengthen. Exhale and relax your shoulders. Gently rocking your body from side to side will continue to loosen the deltoid muscles.

Traditional Asanas: Spread Leg Stretched Out Pose C (Prasarita Padottanasana C)

Filler-up Asana II

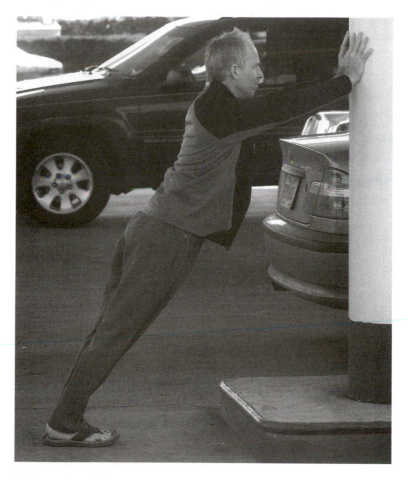

Filler-up Asana II

Time Required: 0 minutes

Benefit: lengthened calf muscles, aides in bending forward

Difficulty: 1

Muscles Awakened: gastrocnemius, soleus

Description: Face a sturdy pole, gas pump, or your vehicle and root down firmly through the four corners of your feet (located in the inner and outer edges of the heels and the base of the big toe and little toe joints in the balls of your feet). Lean forward, placing your hand against the object, your heels remaining on the ground. Gently lift your toes to deepen the stretch. As you breathe, feel your calf muscles relax just a bit more on each exhalation. You will want to find a balance for how far back you place your feet. Locating them too far back will create too much tension in your calves and Achilles tendon. Placing them too far forward will not achieve the optimal amount of stretch that you could gain from this posture.

Traditional Asanas: Downward Facing Dog Pose (Adho Mukha Svanasana)

Variations: Alternately bending each knee slightly will put more pressure in the opposite leg, giving it more of a stretch.

Shopping has always been difficult for me, especially when it is a trip for someone else and I spend considerable time waiting. Once again, we can transform this into an opportunity to do yoga.

Walking can become a meditation and an opportunity for union, or yoga, as I described at the outset. Waiting can be a moment of body awareness, a time to review our posture and how we are standing.

Shopping

Waiting Asana

It is easy for us to be unaware of our bodies while waiting in line. We often are frustrated at having to wait and begin to think about where we should be going next. We worry about something, or perhaps we just feel tired.

When we are unaware of our bodies, we tend to stand in postures which strain our muscles. We might not ground firmly in our feet, we may be putting undue strain on our knees. We may allow our pelvis to tip forward, backward, or to one side, and compressing discs between our vertebrae.

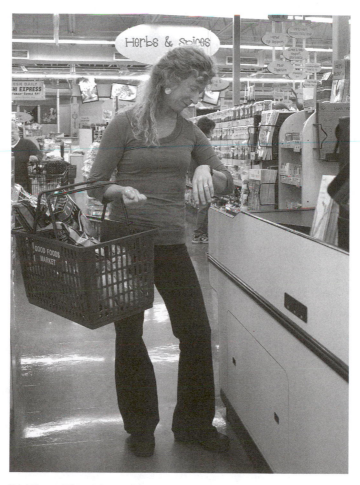

Waiting without intention

An alternative is to remain conscious of our body posture from the balls of our feet all the way up to the crown of our head. For starters, here we notice that our model has placed the groceries on the belt to relieve stress on her body. She is firmly rooted in her feet, standing upright, and comfortable but not rigid. She aligns her hips, pelvis, shoulders, neck, and head very well.

Time Required: 0 minutes

Benefit: improved posture and presence

Difficulty: 1

Muscles Awakened: all muscles used to stand

Description: As you stand in line, set your intention toward caring for your body in that moment. Root down firmly into your feet, wiggle your toes, and sway back and forth a bit. Hold your feet straight, pointing forward, knees open and unlocked. Inhale and breathe into your hips and pelvis. Feel your lower abdomen expand and receive the gift of prana. Exhale and relax your abdominal wall back, offering support for your lower back. Inhale and feel your chest expand outward in all directions. Exhale and relax. Inhale and feel your spine lengthen, your throat gently back and on top of your spine. Exhale and relax. Continue breathing and maintaining awareness of the expansion of your entire body. Make this a meditation in standing. Feel each breath as well as your sense of being alive and connected to everyone and everything around you.

Traditional Asanas: Equal Standing Pose or Mountain Pose (Samasthiti or Tadasana)

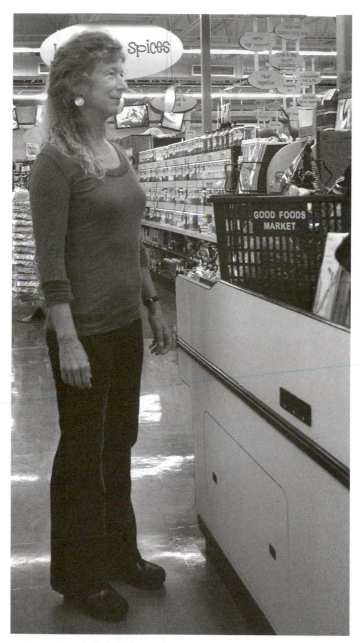

Waiting Asana, with intention

Anywhere

Meditating on Each Moment

As you move through your daily life, you can choose to move through it with little awareness, like a hamster on an exercise wheel, or you can choose to be awake and aware.

Similarly, as you practice the postures in this book you may begin to perceive both subtle and profound physical and emotional feelings in your body, and ultimately, you may become more aware of your behavior patterns. Yoga, or union, will happen if you truly practice. The physical exercises will first bring about physical awareness, then emotional and behavioral awareness, which will bring you closer to a point of stillness, peace, and a deeper part of yourself.

One of the most powerful ways to reach this inner expanse of peace is to bring awareness of everything going on around you at each instant in time. Savor it and make it a moment of meditation.

The present moment is all that we have. The past is gone and cannot be changed. The future has not happened yet, and there is no point in fretting about what may happen in the next minute, day, month, or year. Simply think to yourself: I can never repeat this moment and I have only a finite number of moments to experience in my life. Why not enjoy this moment…and this moment?

At the most elemental level our lives are nothing more than a linear set of experiences. The experiences range from traumatic to blissful. Once each experience has passed, it is no longer alive, it is dead. So we must experience and savor each moment as it is and then let go of it.

In my view, our universe and all that is in it is simply multiple manifestations of an energy which is constantly moving forward like a river. Imagine this river of energy flowing forward in time. We are fully immersed in this river, not just wading. We can cling to branches hanging from the shore and attempt to maintain stability with what is familiar in our lives, but as they say on *Star Trek*, resistance is futile. Let go and enjoy the journey.

If you can embrace this energetic paradigm as you attempt each posture and set your intention of living each moment to its fullest, you can fully enter the energetic flow. Feeling your immersion in the flow allows you to embrace the love and joy present in each moment.

Contribute a Pose

I would like this book to be dynamic and alive. I invite you to write to me at joel@jdigirolamo.com with suggestions for new poses. At a minimum, please send me a description of the pose, but preferably a picture of the pose as well.

If I choose to include your submission in my next edition I will acknowledge you as the creator and will send you a free copy of the first edition with that pose in it. So get that creative kundalini energy flowing!

Table of Difficulty Levels and Time

Sorted by Time

No Time At All

Armpit Scrub Asana
Brush Asana
Brushing Forward Dog Asana
Brushing Pigeon Asana
Chair Asana I
Chair Asana II
Chair Asana III
Chair Asana IV
Chair Asana V
Dishwashing Asana
Dishwashing Tree Asana
Filler-up Asana I
Filler-up Asana II
Pet Asana I
Pet Asana II
Phone Asana
Pick It Out Asana I
Pick It Out Asana II
Revolved Brush Asana
Revolved Chair Asana III
Shave Asana
Shoe Tie Asana
Sleep Asana I
Sleep Asana II
Sock Asana
Stoplight Asana
Waiting Asana

Less Than Three Minutes

Chair Asana VI
Grounding Asana
Neck Tilt Asana I
Neck Tilt Asana II
Neck Tilt Asana III
Prayer Asana
The Rack Asana
Towel Asana

Three to Five Minutes

Bed Asana I
Bed Asana II
Bed Asana III

Sorted by Difficulty

One

Armpit Scrub Asana
Bed Asana I
Bed Asana II
Brush Asana
Brushing Forward Dog Asana
Chair Asana V
Chair Asana VI
Dishwashing Asana
Filler-up Asana II
Grounding Asana
Neck Tilt Asana I
Neck Tilt Asana II
Neck Tilt Asana III
Pet Asana I
Prayer Asana
Sleep Asana II
Stoplight Asana
Waiting Asana

Two

Bed Asana III
Chair Asana I
Chair Asana II

Dishwashing Tree Asana
Sleep Asana I
Shoe Tie Asana
Towel Asana

Three

Brushing Pigeon Asana
Chair Asana III
Filler-up Asana I
Pick It Out Asana I
Pick It Out Asana II
Revolved Chair Asana III
Sock Asana
The Rack Asana

Four

Chair Asana IV
Pet Asana II
Phone Asana
Revolved Brush Asana

Five

Shave Asana

Balancing Poses

Armpit Scrub Asana
Dishwashing Tree Asana
Pet Asana I
Pet Asana II

Phone Asana
Pick It Out Asana II
Shoe Tie Asana
Sock Asana

References

Bachman, N. (2005). *The Language of Yoga: Complete A to Y Guide to Asana Names, Sanskrit Terms, and Chants.* Boulder, CO: Sounds True.

Coulter, H. D. (2001). *Anatomy of Hatha Yoga: A Manual for Students, Teachers, and Practitioners.* Honesdale, PA: Body and Breath, Inc.

Hewitt, J. (1977). *The Complete Yoga Book: Yoga of Breathing, Yoga of Posture, and Yoga of Meditation.* New York: Schocken Books.

Iyengar, B. K. S. (1979). *Light on Yoga: Yoga Dipika.* New York: Schocken Books.

Kaminoff, L. (2007). *Yoga Anatomy.* Champaign, IL: Human Kinetics.

Kapit, W. & Elson, L. M. (1993). *The Anatomy Coloring Book.* New York: HarperCollins College Publishers.

Long, R. (2006). *The Key Muscles of Hatha Yoga.* Bandha Yoga Publications.

Muktibodhananda, S. (1998). *Hatha Yoga Pradipika: Light on Hatha Yoga.* Munger, Bihar, India: Yoga Publications Trust.

Saraswati, S. S. (1996). *Asana Pranayama Mudra Bandha.* Munger, Bihar, India: Yoga Publications Trust.

Sieg, K. W. & Adams, S. P. (1996). *Illustrated Essentials of Musculoskeletal Anatomy.* Gainesville, FL: Megabooks.

Sparrowe, L. & Martinez, D. (2002). *Yoga (Yoga Journal)*. Hugh Lauter Levin Associates, Inc.

Svatmarama. (2002). *The Hatha Yoga Pradipika (B. D. Akers, Trans.)*. Woodstock, NY: YogaVidya.com.

Swenson, D. (1999). Ashtanga Yoga: *The Practice Manual*. Austin, TX: Ashtanga Yoga Productions.

Yesudian, S. & Haich, E. (1953). *Yoga and Health: How to Achieve and Maintain Radiant Health by Correct Breathing and Exercise*. New York: Harper & Brothers.

Glossary of Anatomical Parts

Achilles tendon: a tendon on the lower calf connecting the gastrocnemius and soleus muscles to the heel (calcaneus).

Adductors: a group of muscles that work to bring the legs together.

Anterior superior iliac spine (ASIS): the most forward point of the ilium, or upper portion of the pelvis. Also known as the hip points. These points are very useful to gauge the rotation of your pelvis.

Biceps: a muscle connecting the scapula and radius which works to flex the elbow.

Cervical spine: the upper seven vertebrae of the spine. Commonly referred to as the neck.

Coccyx: see tailbone.

Crown: the top of the head.

Deltoids: a group of three muscles that work to move the arm forward, backward, and away from the body (abduction).

Erector spinae: muscles of the back that work to extend, or flatten the back.

Femur: the large, sturdy, weight-bearing upper leg bone. Bipedal creatures require these large bones since the body weight is carried through two bones as opposed to four in quadrupeds.

Fibula: the lower leg bones, the fibula and tibia, carry the weight of the body and work together to allow rotation, flexion, and extension of the foot and ankle.

Gastrocnemius: a muscle of the calf that works to flex the knee and point, or extend, the foot. The gastrocnemius and soleus both tie in to the Achilles tendon.

Gluteus maximus: the large muscle of the buttocks that works to extend and externally rotate the leg.

Gluteus medius: a muscle underneath the gluteus maximus that works to abduct (move apart) and internally rotate the leg.

Gluteus minimus: a muscle underneath the gluteus medius that works to abduct (move apart) and internally rotate the leg.

Hamstrings: a group of muscles at the back of the leg that work to flex the knee and internally rotate the foot.

Humerus: the upper arm bone.

Infraspinatus: a muscle that works to externally rotate the upper arm.

Internal obliques: an abdominal muscle that works to bring its opposite shoulder forward and twist the chest.

Ischial tuberosity: the lowest point of the pelvic girdle. These are the points of the pelvis that the body rests on when seated on the floor or a chair. Also known as the sitting bones.

Latissimus dorsi: a large sheet of muscles on the back which work to pull the arm down. Also known as the lats.

Lumbar spine: the five lowest vertebrae of the spine. Also known as the lower back.

Pectineus: an adductor muscle that works to flex the upper leg, provide internal rotation, and bring the legs together.

Pectoralis: a group of muscles that work to pull the arms together.

Pelvis: a bowl-shaped set of bones that support the body weight and upward force of the legs. The pelvis provides an attachment point for many muscles of the legs and back.

Piriformis: a muscle that works to rotate the upper leg outward.

Quadriceps: a group of four muscles on the top of the thigh that work to extend the lower leg. Also called quads.

Radius: the forearm bones, the radius and ulna, work together to allow rotation, flexion, and extension of the wrists, hands, and fingers.

Rotator cuff: a group of shoulder muscles. In order for the shoulder joint to allow high mobility it must have a shallow socket. Tension provided by the rotator cuff muscles helps maintain the integrity of this joint. The rotator cuff muscles are supraspinatus, infraspinatus, teres minor, and subscapularis.

Sacrum: five fused vertebrae located between the two ilium bones of the pelvic girdle. The ilium-sacrum joint is called the sacroiliac (SI) joint. The sacrum appears as a keystone-type structure between the ilia and supports the lowest vertebra, L5.

Scalenes: a group of muscles that work to provide flexion of the neck.

Scapula: a highly mobile bone on the back providing numerous muscle attachment points which facilitate movement of the arms and shoulders. Also called the shoulder blade or angel wing.

Sitting bones: see ischial tuberosity.

Soleus: a calf muscle attaching to the Achilles tendon which works to point or extend the foot.

Sternocleidomastoid (SCM): a group of neck muscles that work to flex the neck and tilt the head.

Sternum: the bone at the front of the chest which connects most of the ribs.

Subscapularis: a rotator cuff muscle that works to internally rotate the upper arm.

Tailbone: four small rudimentary vertebrae under the sacrum, constituting the lowest portion of the spine. Also known as the coccyx.

Tensor fasciae latae (TFL): a muscle that works to internally rotate the upper leg and extend the lower leg.

Thoracic spine: the middle 12 vertebrae of the spine.

Tibia: the lower leg bones, the tibia and fibula, carry the weight of the body and work together to allow rotation, flexion, and extension of the foot and ankle.

Trapezius: a sheet of muscles on the upper back that assist body movement by working to bring the scapula upward, downward, and together. Also called the traps.

Triceps: a group of three muscles that work to extend the elbow.

Ulna: the forearm bones, the ulna and radius, work together to allow rotation, flexion, and extension of the wrists, hands, and fingers.

Index

A

Achilles tendon, 25, 120, 137, 138, 139

adductors, 51, 52, 137

Adho Mukha Svanasana, 25, 95, 115, 120

Anterior Superior Iliac Spine (ASIS), 70, 137

Anusara Yoga, 7

Ardha Baddha Padmottanasana, 64, 81

Ardha Baddha Padma Pascimottanasana, 27, 64, 81

Ardha Matsyendrasana, 30

Arm Pressure Pose, 18

Armpit Scrub Asana, 32, 133, 134

asana, 6, 7, 13, 14, 18, 23, 29, 35, 47, 71, 98, 116

Ashtanga Yoga, 7, *see also* **Astanga Yoga**

Astanga Yoga, 7, *see also* **Ashtanga Yoga**

B

Backbend, 39, 54, 115

Baddha Konasana, 27, 51, 52, 81, 83

Balasana, 76

Bed Asana I, 47, 133, 134

Bed Asana II, 48, 133, 134

Bed Asana III, 50, 133, 134

Bhakti Yoga, 6

Bhuja Pidasana, 18

biceps, 35, 137

Big Toe Pose, 18, 64

Bikram Yoga, 7

Bound Angle Pose, 27, 51, 52, 81, 83

Brush Asana, 21, 22, 23, 28, 31, 133, 134

Brushing Forward Dog Asana, 9, 24, 133, 134

Brushing Pigeon Asana, 26, 133, 134

C

cakra, 6, *see also* **chakra**

calf, 25, 81, 89, 119, 120, 137, 138, 139

cervical spine, 41, 64, 93, 137

Chair Asana I, 80, 133, 134

Chair Asana II, 82, 133, 134

Chair Asana III, 84, 133, 134

Chair Asana IV, 88, 133, 134

Chair Asana V, 90, 133, 134

Chair Asana VI, 92, 133, 134

Chair Pose, 33

chakra, 6, *see also* cakra
Child Pose, 76
computer, 9, 100, 102, 104
Cow Face Pose, 35, 54

D
Dancer Pose, 70
deltoids, 29, 33, 41, 53, 115, 117,137
Dishwashing Asana, 57, 133, 134
Dishwashing Tree Asana, 59, 133, 134
Downward Facing Dog Pose, 25, 95, 115, 120
Drive Asana, 113

E
Eagle Pose, 89
enlightenment, 6
Equal Standing Pose, 23, 58, 124
erector spinae, 33, 49, 53, 63, 67, 73, 85, 87, 94, 137
ergonomics, 100
Extended Side Angle Pose, 30
Extended Triangle Pose, 30

F
feet, four corners of, 23, 29, 35, 46, 60, 64, 70, 119
Fierce Pose, 33
Filler-up Asana I, 117, 133, 134
Filler-up Asana II, 119, 133, 134
Foot Hand Pose, 18, 64

G
Garudasana, 89
gastrocnemius, 25, 63, 65, 67, 73, 119, 137, 138
Gentle Yoga, 7

gluteus maximus, 17, 29, 45, 49, 85, 87, 94, 138
gluteus medius, 89, 138
gluteus minimus, 138
Go Mukhasana, 35, 54
Grounding Asana, 94, 96, 104, 109, 133, 134

H
Half Bound Lotus Back Stretched Out Pose, 27, 64, 81
Half Bound Lotus Stretched Out Pose, 64, 81
Half Fish Lord Pose, 30
hamstrings, 17, 18, 60, 63, 65, 67, 94, 138
Hatha Yoga, 6, 7, 135, 136
Hero Pose, 76

I
infraspinatus, 35, 39, 138, 139
intention, 3, 4, 5, 6, 8, 13, 15, 18, 21, 22, 23, 47, 51, 55, 57, 58, 61, 72, 73, 74, 81, 95, 98, 113, 123, 124, 125, 129
internal obliques, 29, 87, 138
ischial tuberosity, 39, 138, 139
Iyengar Yoga, 7

J
Janu Sirsasana, 51, 52
Jivamukti Yoga, 7
Jnana Yoga, 6

K
Karma Yoga, 6
keyboard, 9, 79, 100, 101, 102
Knee Head Pose, 51, 52
Kundalini, 6

Kundalini Yoga, 6
Kurmasana, 18, 95

L
latissimus dorsi, 29, 33, 35, 39, 53, 115, 138
Lord of the Dance Pose, 70
Lord Shiva's Dance Pose, 70
Lotus Pose, 27, 81, 83
lumbar spine, 23, 35, 138

M
Mantra Yoga, 6
Marichyasana, *see* Maricyasana
Maricyasana, 14, 18, 30, 66, 74, 85, 87, 89, 95
meditation, 3, 6, 7, 23, 55, 58, 121, 124, 129, 135
Millimeter Theory, 10, 14
Monkey Mind, 5, 23
Mountain Pose, 23, 58, 124

N
Natarajasana, 70
Neck Tilt Asana I, 97
Neck Tilt Asana II, 99
Neck Tilt Asana III, 99
Noose Pose, 66, 74

O
Oblique Face One Leg Back Stretched Out Pose, 76
obliques, 29, 87, 138

P
Pada Hastasana, 18, 64
Padangusthasana, 18, 64
Padmasana, 27, 81, 83
Parivrtta Parsvakonasana, 30

Parivrtta Trikonasana, 30
Pasasana, 66, 74
Paschimottanasana, 64
pectineus, 27, 81, 83, 138
pectoralis, 29, 33, 35, 39, 41, 53, 70, 115, 117, 138
pelvis, 23, 29, 30, 35, 41, 54, 58, 66, 70, 123, 124, 137, 138
Pet Asana I, 63, 104, 108, 133, 134
Pet Asana II, 65, 104, 108, 133, 134
Phone Asana, 69, 71, 104, 107, 133, 134
Pick It Out Asana I, 72, 73, 133, 134
Pick It Out Asana II, 75, 133, 134
piriformis, 63, 67, 89, 138
Power Yoga, 7
prana, 7, 8, 47, 58, 124
pranayama, 8, 135
Prasarita Padottanasana, 41, 64, 118
Prayer Asana, 38, 104, 105, 133, 134

Q
quadriceps, 29, 47, 60, 64, 68, 70, 74, 75, 89, 138
quads, *see* quadriceps

R
Rack Asana, 40, 104, 106, 133, 134
Raja Yoga, 6
repetitive strain injury (RSI) 79
Revolved Brush Asana, 28, 31, 133, 134
Revolved Chair Asana III, 86, 133, 134
Revolved Side Angle Pose, 30
Revolved Triangle Pose, 30
rotator cuff, 139

S

Sage Marici Pose, 18, 30, 66, 74, 85, 87, 89, 95

samadhi, 6

Samasthiti, 23, 58, 124

scalenes, 97, 99, 139

scapula, 79, 81, 93, 137, 139, 140

SCM, 97, 99, 139

Shave Asana, 17, 19, 20, 133, 134

Shoe Tie Asana, 67, 133, 134

Side Angle Pose, *see* **Extended Side Angle Pose** *or* **Revolved Side Angle Pose**

sitting bones, 39, 81, 83, 85, 87, 94, 98, 99, 138, 139

Sleep Asana I, 52, 133, 134

Sleep Asana II, 53, 133, 134

Sock Asana, 45, 133, 134

soleus, 25, 63, 65, 67, 73, 119, 137, 138

sternocleidomastoid (SCM), 97, 99, 139

Stoplight Asana, 114, 133, 134

subscapularis, 35, 39, 139

Sun Salutation, 33

Surya Namaskara, 33

T

Tadasana, 23, 58, 124

Tantra Yoga, 6

tennis ball, 91

tensor fasciae latae (TFL), 27, 81, 83, 139

TFL, 27, 81, 83, 139

thoracic spine, 64, 139

Three Limbs Face One Foot Western Intense Stretch Pose, 76

Tiryan Mukhaikapada Paschimottanasana, 76

Tortoise Pose, 18, 95

Towel Asana, 34, 36, 37, 133, 134

translate (top of the throat or head), 98, 102. 118

translation, *see* **translate**

trapezius, 35, 99, 140

Tree Pose, 60

Trianga Mukhaikapada Paschimottanasana, 76

Triangle Pose, *see* **Extended Triangle Pose** *or* **Revolved Triangle Pose**

triceps, 29, 33, 35, 39, 53, 70, 140

Trikonasana, *see* **Parivrtta Trikonasana** *or* **Utthita Trikonasana**

U

Upward Bow Pose, 39, 54, 115

Urdhva Dhanurasana, 39, 54, 115

Utkatasana, 33

Uttanasana, 64

Utthita Parsvakonasana, 30

Utthita Trikonasana, 30

V

vinyasa, 7

Virabhadrasana, 33

Virasana, 76

Vrksasana, 60

W

Waiting Asana, 123, 125, 133, 134

Warrior Pose, 33

Wheel Pose, 39, 54, 115

witness state, 9

workstation ergonomics, 100

Y

Yantra Yoga, 6

About the Author

Joel DiGirolamo began practicing yoga at age 12 when his grandfather died. It was at this time that he discovered the book *Yoga and Health* by Selvarajan Yesudian and Elisabeth Haich at his grandfather's house. True to the cycle of death and rebirth, the death of his grandfather gave birth to Joel's spiritual and physical awakening.

At this early age he mastered yoga poses using only this book for guidance and continued practicing by himself on and off over the years. In 2005 he began an Astanga (Ashtanga) Yoga practice in a classroom setting and currently instructs beginning Astanga Yoga students. He is working on his yoga teacher training certificate and maintains a personal daily yoga practice.

While working in the corporate realm much of his day, he became curious as to how he could further incorporate yoga into his daily life—and so the idea of this book was born.